Delicious
Diabetes
C O O K B O O K
BOOK 2

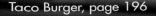

Taco Burger, page 196

Deep-Dish Cherry Pie, page 56

Delicious
WAYS TO CONTROL
Diabetes
C O O K B O O K
BOOK 2

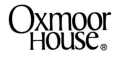

Oxmoor House®

© 2000 by Oxmoor House, Inc.
Book Division of Southern Progress Corporation
P.O. Box 2463, Birmingham, Alabama 35201

ISBN: 0-8487-1968-9
ISSN: 1523-8032
Manufactured in the United States of America
First Printing 2000

Be sure to check with your health-care provider before making any changes in your diet.

Editor-in-Chief: Nancy Fitzpatrick Wyatt
Senior Foods Editor: Katherine M. Eakin
Senior Editor, Copy and Homes: Olivia Kindig Wells
Art Director: James Boone

Delicious Ways to Control Diabetes Cookbook Book 2

Editor: Anne Chappell Cain, M.S., M.P.H., R.D.
Associate Art Director: Cynthia R. Cooper
Designer: Carol O. Loria
Contributing Copy Editor: Shari K. Wimberly
Editorial Assistant: Heather Averett
Medical Advisors: David D. DeAtkine, Jr., M.D.;
    Kris Ernst, R.N., C.D.E.; Cathy A. Wesler, R.D.
Director, Test Kitchens: Elizabeth Tyler Luckett
Assistant Director, Test Kitchens: Julie Christopher
Recipe Editor: Gayle Hays Sadler
Test Kitchens Staff: Gretchen Feldtman, R.D.,
    Natalie E. King, Rebecca W. Mohr, Leigh Mullinax,
    Jan A. Smith, Kate M. Wheeler, R.D.
Senior Photographer: Jim Bathie
Photographer: Brit Huckabay
Additional photography: Ralph Anderson
Senior Photo Stylist: Kay E. Clarke
Photo Stylist: Virginia Cravens
Director, Production and Distribution: Phillip Lee
Associate Production Manager: Theresa L. Beste
Production Assistant: Faye Porter Bonner

We're Here for You!

We at Oxmoor House are dedicated to serving you with reliable information that expands your imagination and enriches your life. We welcome your comments and suggestions. Please write us at:

Oxmoor House, Inc.
Editor, *Delicious Ways to Control Diabetes Cookbook*
2100 Lakeshore Drive
Birmingham, AL 35209

To order additional publications, call 1-205-877-6560. Or if you have diabetic recipes to share, please send them to the above address. Be sure to include your name and daytime telephone number.

Cover: Raspberry-Mocha Cake, page 57

Contents

Dear Friends,

Mealtime should be a pleasant experience of enjoying good food with family and friends. But when you have diabetes, sometimes it seems that meals are more like a prescription than a pleasure. It's true that what you eat affects your blood glucose, but it *is* possible to control your diabetes without giving up the joys of the table.

It's a lovely thing—everyone sitting down together sharing food.

ALICE MAY BROCK, American restaurateur

I'm a dietitian and have had diabetes since I was 12 years old. Mealtime has always been my favorite time, and I don't believe you have to turn a delightful ritual into a diet therapy session.

With Book 2 in the *Delicious Ways to Control Diabetes Cookbook* series, we want to help you enjoy food as you live with diabetes. Our staff of registered dietitians and cooking experts have put together over 100 recipes plus a one-week menu plan so that you and your family can enjoy wonderful meals together without giving up diabetes control. Each recipe has nutrient information and exchanges, so you can work it into your meal plan without worry— whether you are counting carbohydrates or using exchange lists.

Since everybody seems to be pressed for time these days, we've included quick recipes and make-ahead recipes. We've kept the ingredient lists short and the methods simple. We hope the beautiful food photography will inspire you as well as give you an idea of how the prepared recipe will look when you serve it to family and friends.

Welcome, and please join me at the table.

Sincerely,

Anne Cain

Anne Cain, Editor

2000 UPDATE

The Year's Best News for People with Diabetes

*Until there's a cure, here's some of the best news
we've heard this year about diabetes.*

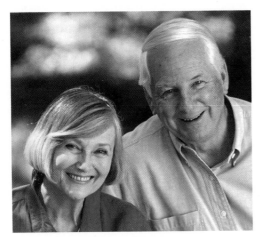

More Care from Medicare

Medicare now pays for insulin pumps for people in the program with Type 1 diabetes. *The new policy applies to only those people with Type 1 who take at least three insulin injections a day and check their blood glucose at least four times a day.*

Medicare now also covers blood glucose testing supplies for people who control diabetes with insulin, diabetes pills, or diet. Medicare pays 80% of the cost of glucose meters, strips, and lancets.

For more specific information about Medicare coverage, call 800-489-4633.

The Promise of a Pill?

A fungus called *Pseudomassaria*, which grows on leaves in the African Congo, yields a compound that acts just like insulin in test-tube cells and in mice with diabetes symptoms. The compound interacts with cell receptors in a way that allows the cells to use and store blood glucose. When the compound was given to mice with diabetes symptoms, the mice had a significant lowering of blood glucose levels.

A great deal more work must be done, however, to find out whether this compound can be developed into a pill that could replace insulin.

Don't get rid of your insulin bottles yet, but there are some talented scientists who believe this compound has great potential for people with diabetes.

Fingertip Freedom

In last year's update, we told you about the development of glucose monitors that did not require finger sticks. Now one has made it to the market: The **AtLast™ Blood Glucose System** (Amira Medical) is available through mail order. This product has an all-in-one lance and metering device, and is used in the forearm, upper arm, or thigh. (These areas have fewer nerve endings than the fingertips, so the tests are less painful.)

Here's how it works: Place a test strip in one end of the meter. Press the other end into the forearm until the system lances the skin. Repeat the "press and release" motion several times to draw a very small amount of blood to the surface of the skin. Turn the meter over and touch the test strip to the blood sample. When the strip has absorbed enough blood (about 2uL) a beep sounds. In 15 seconds the meter displays your blood glucose level.

As this monitor was being tested, 90 percent of the people who used it said that they had significantly less or no pain compared to fingerstick methods. **For more information about AtLast, call 877-264-7263.**

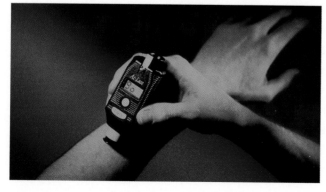

Pen Pals

If you're an insulin-user looking for a little more convenience, an insulin pen may be for you. The devices look like large pens and contain prefilled insulin cartridges and disposable needles. Instead of drawing the correct dose of insulin into a syringe, you select the amount you need with a dial.

Pen Benefits
- easy to carry in a purse or a pocket
- does not need refrigeration
- sturdy
- accurate (because you dial the numbers instead of having to look at the measurement lines on a syringe)
- one device to carry instead of syringes and bottles of insulin

Both Eli Lilly and Company and Novo Nordisk Pharmaceuticals have pens for several types of insulin. **Ask your doctor if a pen would be appropriate for you.**

Watch Out

It's almost here: A wrist-worn device that provides frequent, automatic, noninvasive blood glucose monitoring for adults (18 years and older).

The GlucoWatch (Cygnus, Inc.) extracts a tiny sample of blood through the skin, and the sample is measured by a sensor pad inside the watch. Through an electro-chemical process, the sensor translates the measurement into a blood glucose reading which it displays on the monitor and stores in the memory. Each day, you replace rechargeable batteries and insert a new sensor pad into the monitor. You have to do a finger-stick test to calibrate the monitor and wait three hours for it to warm up. Then the monitor automatically tests blood glucose levels every 20 minutes for the next 12 hours. If levels are too low, an alarm will sound.

A Food and Drug Administration (FDA) advisory committee reviewed the watch in December 1999, but the manufacturers have to wait for final FDA approval before the GlucoWatch will be on the market. **For more information, check out the Cygnus Web site at www.cygn.com or call 650-369-4300.**

V-Day for Diabetes?

Imagine going to the doctor for a vaccination to keep you from getting diabetes. A Canadian diabetes research team led by Dr. Ji-Won Yoon showed that diabetes does not occur in animals if the immune system is prevented from attacking a certain enzyme present in insulin-producing cells. Researchers think that if the immune system is exposed to the enzyme by a vaccine and becomes accustomed to this enzyme (and did not think it was "foreign"), it would not attack the cells and diabetes would not occur.

The studies with animals and nondiabetic people showed that the vaccine is safe. Now the researchers are waiting for approval to conduct more studies. Dr. David Lau, the research director, says, **"We don't have a cure yet but it offers a lot more insight and hope, and we are one step closer to a cure."**

Splendid Splenda

It's sweeter than sugar and calorie-free. It doesn't have a bitter aftertaste. It's heat stable and can be used in baking. It doesn't affect blood glucose levels or promote tooth decay. What is it?

The new sweetener on the market is **sucralose** (brand name: Splenda). Sucralose is the only calorie-free sweetener that is made from sugar through a manufacturing process that changes the sugar molecule and produces a sweetener that is 600 times sweeter than table sugar (sucrose).

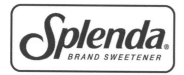

Sucralose is available now as an ingredient in carbonated soft drinks, low-calorie fruit drinks, maple syrup, and applesauce. Look for the name Splenda Brand Sweetener on the label.

By early 2001, Splenda should be available in supermarkets as a tabletop sweetener in granulated form and in packets.

Until then, you can purchase Splenda on the Internet at www.splenda.com.

Round-the-Clock Nutrition Advisor

You can now have access to nutrition information any time you need it through an Internet interactive program called "Treating Diabetes Through Good Nutrition."

This program offers a personalized nutrition profile that helps you determine how many calories you need and then creates 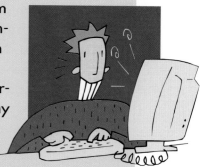 a meal plan. Learn about nutrition topics such as counting carbohydrates, using exchange lists, eating out, and using sweeteners. You can also find new recipes and learn how to modify your old ones for your health needs. Among the program's best features are the Weekly Menu Plans (plus grocery lists) for your specific calorie level.

To find the Web site, go to www.cyberdiet.com and click on "Treating Diabetes."

While this Web site does not replace the benefits of personal counseling with a registered dietitian, it does offer accurate, helpful information whenever you need it.

Appetizers & Beverages

Spicy Tortilla Chips, page 18
and Fiesta Onion Salsa, page 14

Creamy Pineapple Dip • Fiesta Onion Salsa • Hot Crabmeat Dip
Spicy Snack Mix • Spicy Tortilla Chips • Marinated Cheese Appetizers
Mexican Pinwheels • Citrus Punch • Watermelon-Berry Slush
Spicy Tomato Sipper

Creamy Pineapple Dip

Yield: 1¼ cups

1   cup lemon low-fat yogurt sweetened with aspartame
3   tablespoons frozen pineapple juice concentrate
1   tablespoon fat-free sour cream

Combine all ingredients in a small bowl; stir well. Cover and chill at least 25 minutes.

Stir just before serving. Serve with assorted fresh fruit (fruit not included in analysis).

Store remaining dip in an airtight container in the refrigerator up to 5 days.

Per Tablespoon:

Calories 22	Fiber 0.0g
Fat 0.1g (sat 0.1g)	Cholesterol 0mg
Protein 0.5g	Sodium 9mg
Carbohydrate 4.7g	Exchange: Free (up to 2 tablespoons)

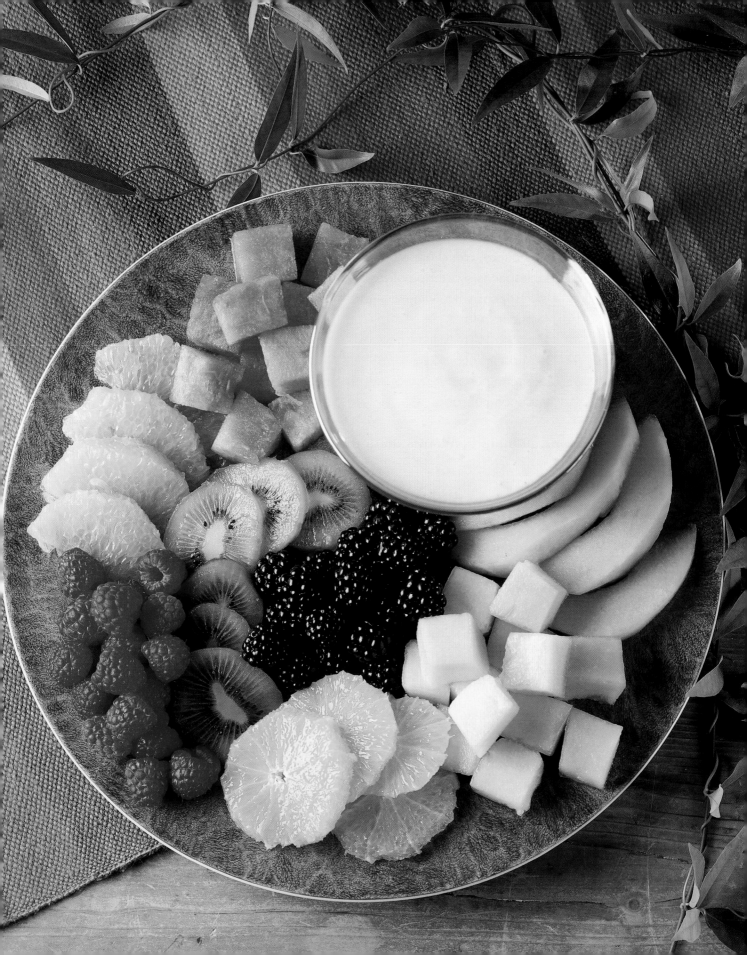

Fiesta Onion Salsa

Yield: 2 cups

1	cup chopped onion (about 1 large)
¾	cup chopped tomato (about 1 medium)
1	(4.5-ounce) can chopped green chiles, drained
3	tablespoons sliced ripe olives
2	tablespoons white wine vinegar
¼	teaspoon salt
¼	teaspoon Worcestershire sauce
⅛	teaspoon ground cumin
⅛	teaspoon pepper
⅛	teaspoon hot sauce

Combine all ingredients in a medium bowl; cover and chill at least 2 hours.

Serve with low-fat tortilla chips (chips not included in analysis).

Per Tablespoon:

Calories 5	Fiber 0.2g
Fat 0.2g (sat 0.0g)	Cholesterol 0mg
Protein 0.1g	Sodium 45mg
Carbohydrate 0.9g	Exchange: Free

(Photograph on page 11)

This salsa is also great on grilled chicken and fish.

Hot Crabmeat Dip

Yield: 3½ cups

2	(8-ounce) ⅓-less-fat cream cheese (Neufchâtel)
½	cup nonfat mayonnaise
¼	cup grated onion
½	teaspoon garlic powder
¼	teaspoon salt
½	teaspoon pepper
3	tablespoons dry white wine
2	teaspoons prepared mustard
2	teaspoons prepared horseradish
½	pound fresh lump crabmeat, drained
2	tablespoons chopped fresh chives
2	tablespoons chopped fresh parsley

Combine first 9 ingredients in a medium saucepan, stir well. Cook over low heat, stirring constantly, until cream cheese melts and mixture is smooth.

Stir in crabmeat and remaining ingredients. Transfer to a chafing dish, and keep warm.

Serve with low-fat crackers (crackers not included in analysis).

Per Tablespoon:

Calories 25	**Fiber** 0.1g
Fat 1.5g (sat 0.8g)	**Cholesterol** 9mg
Protein 1.7g	**Sodium** 97mg
Carbohydrate 1.2g	**Exchange:** Free (up to 4 tablespoons)

Spicy Snack Mix

Yield: 10 (½-cup) servings

1½ cups bite-size crispy corn squares
1½ cups bite-size crispy rice squares
1½ cups bite-size crispy wheat squares
¾ cup small unsalted pretzels
¼ cup unsalted dry roasted peanuts
¼ cup fat-free margarine, melted
2 tablespoons low-sodium soy sauce
1½ teaspoons chili powder
½ teaspoon garlic powder
¼ teaspoon ground red pepper

Combine first 5 ingredients in a large heavy-duty, zip-top plastic bag. Combine margarine and remaining 4 ingredients; pour over cereal mixture. Seal bag; shake well to coat.

Place cereal mixture in a 15- x 10-inch jellyroll pan. Bake at 300° for 18 to 20 minutes, stirring occasionally. Remove from oven; let cool completely.

Store snack mix in an airtight container.

Per Serving:

Calories 59	Fiber 0.6g
Fat 0.6g (sat 0.1g)	Cholesterol 0mg
Protein 1.3g	Sodium 223mg
Carbohydrate 11.6g	Exchange: 1 Starch

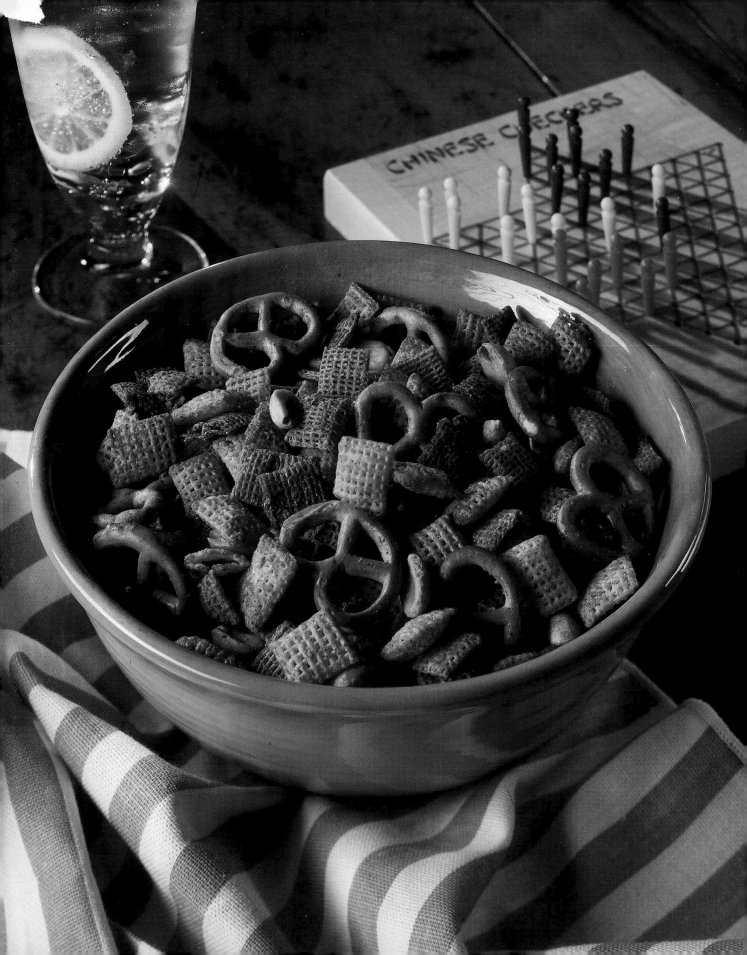

Spicy Tortilla Chips

Yield: 12 servings (serving size: 4 chips)

12   (6-inch) corn tortillas
½   cup lime juice
¼   cup water
½   teaspoon garlic powder
¼   teaspoon salt
⅛   teaspoon ground cumin
⅛   teaspoon ground red pepper

Cut each tortilla into 4 wedges. Combine lime juice and water. Dip wedges in lime juice mixture; drain on paper towels. Arrange wedges in a single layer on a large baking sheet.

Combine garlic powder and remaining 3 ingredients; sprinkle evenly over wedges.

Bake at 350° for 12 to 14 minutes or until crisp. Transfer chips to wire racks; cool completely.

Store chips in an airtight container.

Per Serving:

Calories 60	**Fiber** 1.3g
Fat 0.6g (sat 0.1g)	**Cholesterol** 0mg
Protein 1.5g	**Sodium** 89mg
Carbohydrate 12.7g	**Exchange:** 1 Starch

(Photograph on page 11)

Make Ahead!

Marinated Cheese Appetizers

Yield: 44 appetizers

1   (8-ounce) block part-skim mozzarella cheese
1   (8-ounce) block reduced-fat Cheddar cheese
1   cup fat-free Italian salad dressing
¼   teaspoon freshly ground pepper
1   (12-ounce) French baguette
Fresh basil leaves (optional)

Cut cheeses into ¼-inch-thick slices; place slices in a 13- x 9-inch dish, overlapping slightly.

Combine dressing and pepper; pour over cheese. Cover and chill 8 hours.

Cut baguette into ¼-inch slices. Place on baking sheets. Bake at 350° for 8 to 10 minutes or until lightly toasted, turning once.

Drain cheeses. Place 1 cheese slice on each bread slice. Garnish with fresh basil, if desired.

Per Appetizer:

Calories 52	Fiber 0.1g
Fat 2.0g (sat 1.2g)	Cholesterol 7mg
Protein 3.5g	Sodium 163mg
Carbohydrate 5.2g	Exchange: ½ Medium-Fat Meat

To make ahead, marinate the cheese overnight in the refrigerator. Toast the bread a day ahead, and store it at room temperature. Assemble the appetizers right before serving.

Mexican Pinwheels

Yield: 32 servings (serving size: 2 pinwheels)

1   (8-ounce) package fat-free cream cheese, softened
½   cup fat-free sour cream
1   cup (4 ounces) shredded reduced-fat sharp Cheddar cheese
⅓   cup chopped green onions
¼   teaspoon salt-free herb-and-spice blend
1   (4.5-ounce) can chopped green chiles, drained
1   (2¼-ounce) can sliced ripe olives, drained
1   clove garlic, pressed
8   (8-inch) flour tortillas

Beat cream cheese and sour cream at medium speed of an electric mixer until smooth. Stir in Cheddar cheese and next 5 ingredients. Spread cheese mixture evenly over each tortilla; roll up tortillas. Wrap each separately in plastic wrap. Chill up to 8 hours.

To serve, unwrap each roll, and cut into 8 slices. Secure pinwheels with wooden picks, if desired.

Per Serving:

Calories 52	Fiber 0.4g
Fat 1.6g (sat 0.5g)	Cholesterol 4mg
Protein 3.1g	Sodium 181mg
Carbohydrate 6.0g	Exchange: ½ Starch

Citrus Punch

Yield: 13 (1-cup) servings

4   cups water, divided
3   cups unsweetened pineapple juice
½   cup lemon juice
¼   cup granulated sugar substitute (such as Sugar Twin)
1   (6-ounce) can frozen orange juice concentrate
3   (12-ounce) cans sugar-free lemon-lime carbonated beverage, chilled
Lime slices (optional)

Combine first 5 ingredients in a large bowl; cover and chill.

To serve, stir in carbonated beverage. Serve immediately over ice. Garnish with lime slices, if desired.

Per Serving:

Calories 59	**Fiber** 0.2g
Fat 0.1g (sat 0.0g)	**Cholesterol** 0mg
Protein 0.5g	**Sodium** 19mg
Carbohydrate 14.6g	**Exchange:** 1 Fruit

(Photograph on page 22)

Men and melons are hard to know.

BENJAMIN FRANKLIN

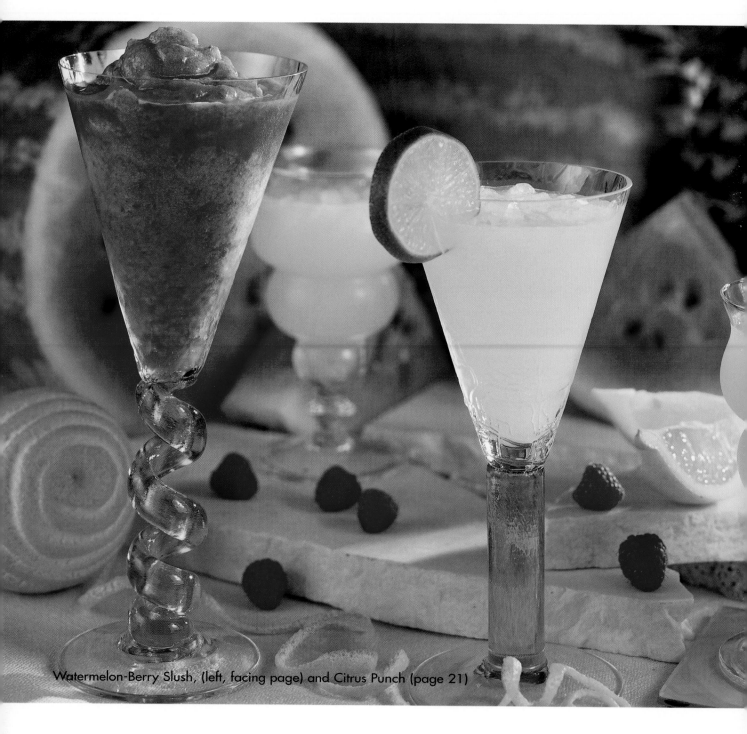

Watermelon-Berry Slush, (left, facing page) and Citrus Punch (page 21)

Watermelon-Berry Slush

Yield: 5 (1-cup) servings

4   cups seeded, cubed watermelon
1   (10-ounce) package frozen raspberries in light syrup
1   (11-ounce) bottle sparkling water

Place watermelon cubes in a single layer in a shallow pan; freeze until firm.

Remove watermelon from freezer; let stand 5 minutes. Position knife blade in food processor bowl. Drop watermelon through food chute with processor running; process until smooth. Add chunks of frozen raspberries alternately with sparkling water; processing until mixture is smooth.

Serve immediately.

Per Serving:

Calories 72	Fiber 2.7g
Fat 0.5g (sat 0.3g)	Cholesterol 0mg
Protein 0.7g	Sodium 18mg
Carbohydrate 16.9g	Exchange: 1 Fruit

Spicy Tomato Sipper

Yield: 3 (1-cup) servings

2¾ cups no-salt-added tomato juice
2 tablespoons lime juice
2 teaspoons low-sodium Worcestershire sauce
1 teaspoon prepared horseradish
½ teaspoon celery salt
¼ teaspoon hot sauce
Lime curls (optional)

Combine first 6 ingredients in a small pitcher; stir well. Cover and chill thoroughly.

Garnish with lime curls, if desired.

Per Serving:

Calories 51	**Fiber** 0.9g
Fat 0.0g (sat 0.0g)	**Cholesterol** 0mg
Protein 2.3g	**Sodium** 390mg
Carbohydrate 12.9g	**Exchanges:** 2 Vegetable

For an even spicier drink, increase the hot sauce to ½ teaspoon.

Breads

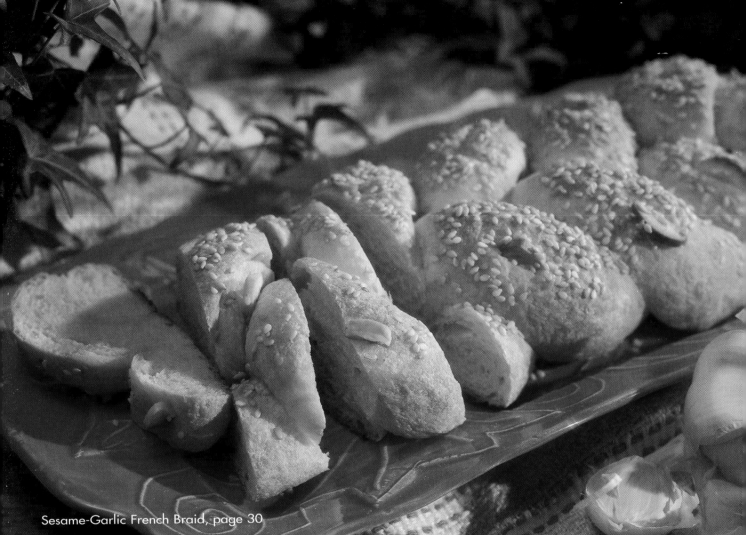

Sesame-Garlic French Braid, page 30

Sour Cream Rolls • Onion-Sesame Rolls • Herbed Garlic Bread
Sesame-Garlic French Braid • Sage and Cheese Biscuits
Whole Wheat Banana Muffins • Overnight Bran Muffins
Cornmeal Muffins • Applesauce Pancakes • Baked Hush Puppies
Spoonbread • Monkey Bread • Quick Yeast Rolls

Sour Cream Rolls

Yield: 1 dozen

2¼ cups reduced-fat biscuit and baking mix, divided
1   (8-ounce) carton fat-free sour cream
½   cup reduced-calorie margarine, melted
Cooking spray

Combine 2 cups biscuit mix, sour cream, and margarine, stirring well.

Sprinkle remaining ¼ cup biscuit mix on a flat surface. Drop dough by level tablespoonfuls onto surface, and roll into balls. Place 3 balls into each of 12 muffin cups coated with cooking spray.

Bake at 350° for 20 minutes or until rolls are golden.

Serve immediately.

Per Roll:

Calories 140	Fiber 0.2g
Fat 6.5g (sat 1.0g)	Cholesterol 0mg
Protein 2.7g	Sodium 345mg
Carbohydrate 17.0g	Exchanges: 1 Starch, 1 Fat

Onion-Sesame Rolls

Yield: 10 rolls

1½ tablespoons grated Parmesan cheese
1 tablespoon instant minced onion
½ teaspoon garlic powder
1 (10-ounce) can refrigerated pizza dough
Butter-flavored cooking spray
2 tablespoons fat-free Italian salad dressing
1 tablespoon sesame seeds

Combine first 3 ingredients; set cheese mixture aside.

Unroll pizza dough, and pat into a 10- x 8-inch rectangle. Coat dough with cooking spray, and brush with salad dressing. Sprinkle cheese mixture over dough, leaving a ½-inch border. Roll up, jellyroll fashion, starting with short side; pinch seams to seal.

Cut into 10 (1-inch-thick) slices, and place on an ungreased baking sheet. Coat tops of rolls with cooking spray, and sprinkle with sesame seeds.

Bake at 400° for 10 to 12 minutes or until rolls are lightly browned.

Serve immediately.

Per Roll:

Calories 87	Fiber 0.5g
Fat 1.9g (sat 0.4g)	Cholesterol 1mg
Protein 3.1g	Sodium 204mg
Carbohydrate 14.4g	Exchange: 1 Starch

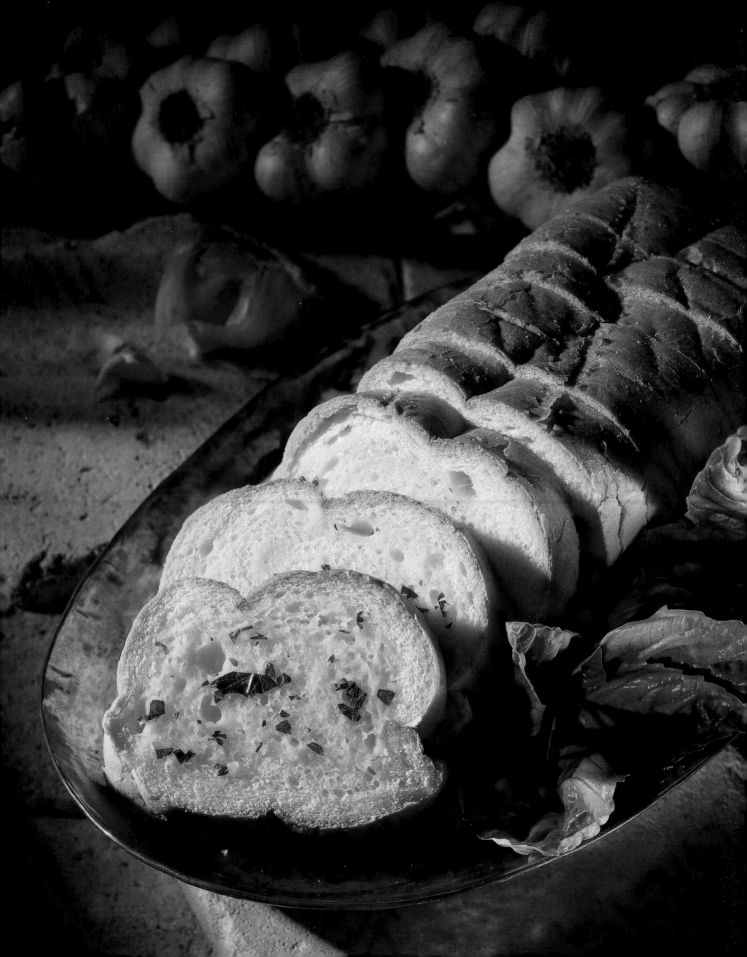

Herbed Garlic Bread

Yield: 12 (¾-inch) slices

¼   cup reduced-calorie margarine, softened
1½ tablespoons freshly grated Parmesan cheese
2   teaspoons minced fresh parsley
2   teaspoons minced fresh basil
¼   teaspoon garlic powder
12   (¾-inch-thick) slices French bread

Combine first 5 ingredients in a small bowl; stir well. Spread mixture evenly on one side of bread slices.

Wrap bread in aluminum foil, and bake at 400° for 15 minutes.

Remove bread from foil, and serve warm.

Per Slice:

Calories 103	**Fiber** 0.7g
Fat 3.0g (sat 0.5g)	**Cholesterol** 1mg
Protein 2.6g	**Sodium** 203mg
Carbohydrate 15.8g	**Exchanges:** 1 Starch, ½ Fat

Get the flavor of commercial garlic bread but a lot less fat with plain French bread and our low-fat cheese-herb mixture.

Sesame-Garlic French Braid

Yield: 10 servings

1   (11-ounce) can refrigerated French bread dough
Cooking spray
2   cloves garlic, thinly sliced
1½   tablespoons reduced-calorie margarine, melted
2   teaspoons sesame seeds

Unroll dough; cut into 3 equal pieces. Shape each portion into a
rope. Place ropes on a baking sheet coated with cooking spray; (do
not stretch). Braid ropes (see photo); pinch loose ends to seal.
Insert garlic slices evenly into braid. Brush melted margarine over
braid, and sprinkle with sesame seeds.

Bake braid at 350° for 25 minutes or until loaf sounds hollow when
tapped. Remove from baking sheet immediately. Serve warm.

Per Serving:

Calories 86	Fiber 0.3g
Fat 2.2g (sat 0.7g)	Cholesterol 0mg
Protein 3.1g	Sodium 212mg
Carbohydrate 13.7g	Exchange: 1 Starch

(Photograph on page 25)

Making a Bread Braid

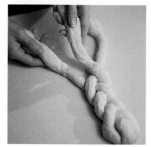

Sage and Cheese Biscuits

Yield: 8 biscuits

1	cup all-purpose flour
1½	teaspoons baking powder
¼	teaspoon salt
1	teaspoon ground sage
⅛	teaspoon freshly ground pepper
2	tablespoons margarine
⅓	cup fat-free evaporated milk
2	tablespoons (½ ounce) shredded reduced-fat Monterey Jack cheese
1½	teaspoons all-purpose flour

Combine first 5 ingredients in a large bowl; cut in margarine with a pastry blender until mixture resembles coarse meal. Add milk and cheese, stirring just until dry ingredients are moistened.

Sprinkle 1½ teaspoons flour over work surface. Turn dough out onto floured surface, and knead 10 to 12 times. Roll dough to ½-inch thickness; cut into rounds using a 2-inch biscuit cutter.

Place rounds on an ungreased baking sheet. Bake at 450° for 8 to 10 minutes or until biscuits are golden.

Serve warm.

Per Biscuit:

Calories 93	Fiber 0.4g
Fat 3.4g (sat 0.8g)	Cholesterol 2mg
Protein 2.8g	Sodium 189mg
Carbohydrate 12.7g	Exchanges: 1 Starch, ½ Fat

Whole Wheat Banana Muffins

Yield: 16 muffins

1   cup all-purpose flour
1   cup whole wheat flour
¼   cup toasted wheat germ
1   teaspoon baking powder
1   teaspoon baking soda
½   teaspoon salt
1½   cups mashed very ripe bananas (about 3 large)
¼   cup sugar
2   tablespoons granulated sugar substitute (such as Sugar Twin)
¼   cup vegetable oil
1   egg, lightly beaten
Cooking spray

Combine first 6 ingredients in a large bowl; make a well in center of mixture.

Combine banana and next 4 ingredients; add to dry ingredients, stirring just until dry ingredients are moistened.

Spoon mixture into muffin pans coated with cooking spray, filling two-thirds full. Bake at 350° for 20 minutes.

Serve warm.

Per Muffin:

Calories 128	Fiber 1.9g
Fat 4.3g (sat 0.6g)	Cholesterol 13mg
Protein 2.7g	Sodium 151mg
Carbohydrate 20.6g	Exchanges: 1 Starch, 1 Fat

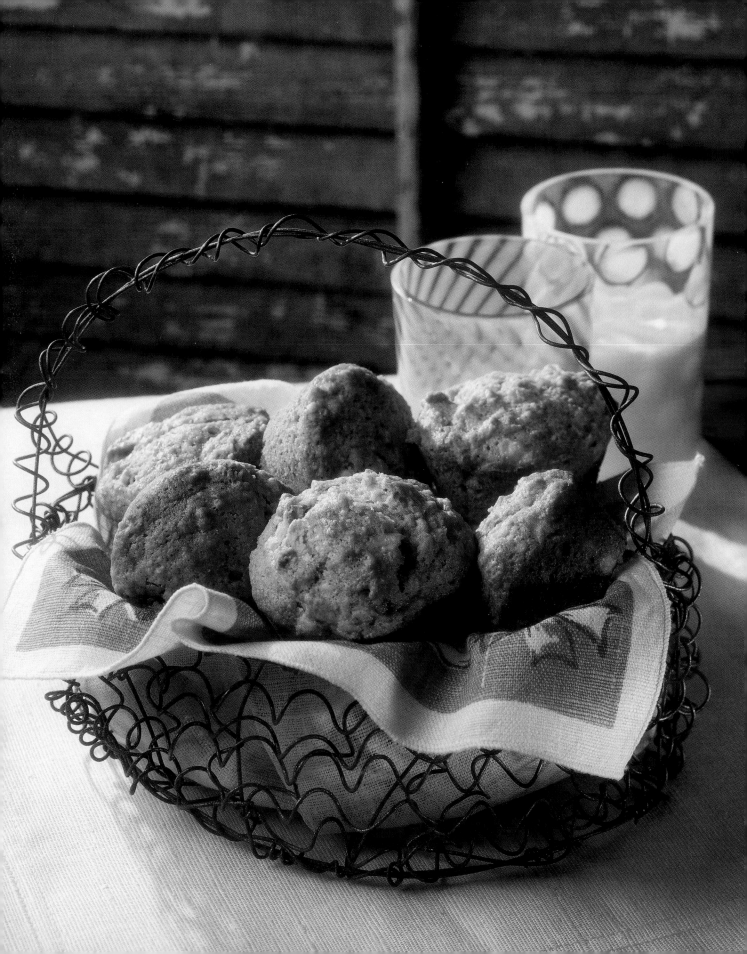

Overnight Bran Muffins

Yield: 2 dozen

4 cups (6 ounces) wheat bran flakes cereal with raisins
2½ cups all-purpose flour
1½ teaspoons baking soda
1 teaspoon salt
1 cup mixed dried fruit
½ cup granulated sugar substitute (such as Sugar Twin)
2 cups nonfat buttermilk
¼ cup corn oil
2 eggs, lightly beaten
Cooking spray

Combine first 6 ingredients in a large bowl; make a well in center of mixture. Combine buttermilk, oil, and eggs; add to dry ingredients, stirring just until dry ingredients are moistened. Cover and chill at least 8 hours.

Spoon batter into muffin pans coated with cooking spray, filling about three-fourths full. Bake at 400° for 14 to 15 minutes or until golden.

Remove muffins from pans immediately, and serve warm.

Per Muffin:

Calories 126	Fiber 1.9g
Fat 3.2g (sat 0.5g)	Cholesterol 18mg
Protein 3.1g	Sodium 227mg
Carbohydrate 22.0g	Exchanges: 1½ Starch, ½ Fat

You can make this muffin batter ahead of time and store it in the refrigerator up to three days.

Cornmeal Muffins

Yield: 1 dozen

1   cup yellow cornmeal
1   cup all-purpose flour
2   teaspoons baking powder
1   teaspoon baking soda
½   teaspoon salt
2   teaspoons granulated sugar substitute (such as Sugar Twin)
1½   cups nonfat buttermilk
¼   cup fat-free egg substitute
3   tablespoons vegetable oil
Cooking spray

Combine first 6 ingredients in a bowl; make a well in center of mixture. Combine buttermilk, egg substitute, and oil; add to dry ingredients, stirring just until dry ingredients are moistened.

Spoon batter into muffin pans coated with cooking spray, filling three-fourths full. Bake at 425° for 14 minutes or until golden.

Remove muffins from pans immediately, and serve warm.

Per Muffin:

Calories 124	Fiber 0.9g
Fat 4.0g (sat 0.7g)	Cholesterol 1mg
Protein 3.6g	Sodium 262mg
Carbohydrate 18.2g	Exchanges: 1 Starch, 1 Fat

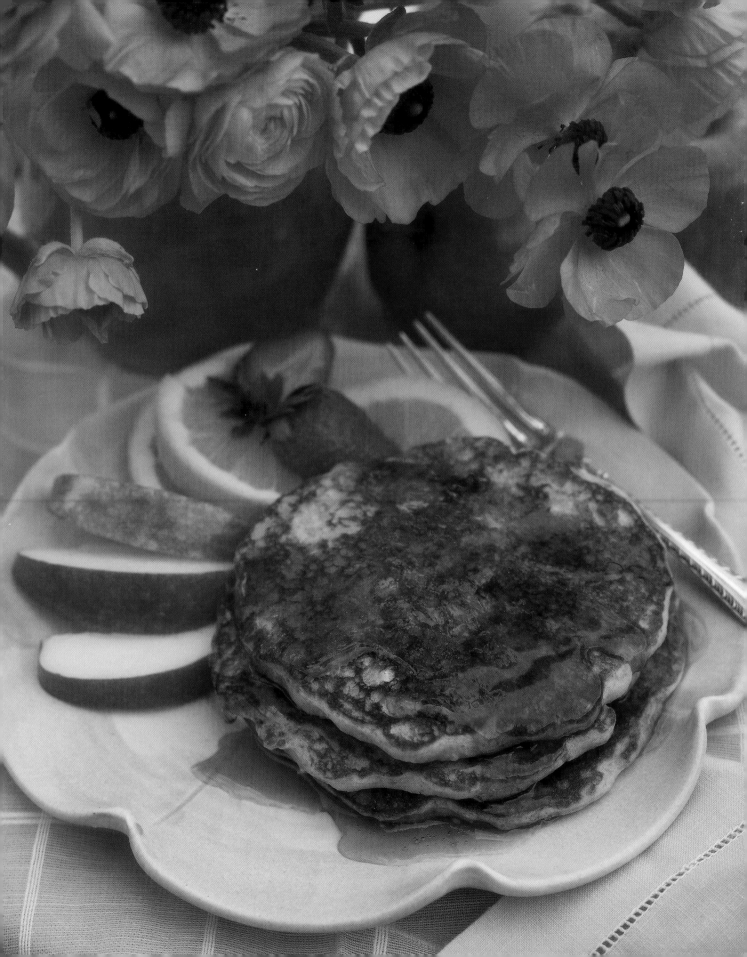

Ready in 20 Minutes!

Applesauce Pancakes

Yield: 10 (5-inch) pancakes

1	cup all-purpose flour
1	teaspoon baking soda
⅛	teaspoon salt
2	tablespoons toasted wheat germ
1	cup nonfat buttermilk
¼	cup unsweetened applesauce
2	teaspoons vegetable oil
1	egg, lightly beaten

Cooking spray
Reduced-calorie maple syrup (optional)
Fresh fruit slices (optional)

Combine first 4 ingredients in a medium bowl; make a well in center of mixture. Combine buttermilk and next 3 ingredients. Add buttermilk mixture to dry ingredients, stirring just until dry ingredients are moistened.

Coat a nonstick griddle or nonstick skillet with cooking spray, and preheat to 350°. For each pancake, pour ¼ cup batter onto hot griddle, spreading to a 5-inch circle. Cook pancakes until tops are covered with bubbles and edges look cooked; turn pancakes, and cook other side.

Serve with maple syrup and fresh fruit, if desired (syrup and fruit not included in analysis).

Per Pancake:

Calories 74	Fiber 0.6g
Fat 1.8g (sat 0.4g)	Cholesterol 22mg
Protein 3.0g	Sodium 143mg
Carbohydrate 11.5g	Exchange: 1 Starch

Baked Hush Puppies

Yield: 3 dozen

1	cup yellow cornmeal
1	cup all-purpose flour
1	tablespoon baking powder
1	teaspoon granulated sugar substitute (such as Sugar Twin)
1	teaspoon salt
1/8	teaspoon ground red pepper
2	eggs, lightly beaten
3/4	cup fat-free milk
1/4	cup vegetable oil
1/2	cup finely chopped onion
Cooking spray	

Combine first 6 ingredients in a large bowl; make a well in center of mixture. Combine eggs and next 3 ingredients, stirring well; add to dry ingredients, stirring just until dry ingredients are moistened.

Coat miniature (1¾-inch) muffin pans with cooking spray. Spoon about 1 tablespoon batter into each muffin cup (cups will be about three-fourths full).

Bake at 425° for 15 minutes or until done. Remove from pans immediately, and serve warm.

Per Hush Puppy:

Calories 56	Fiber 0.4g
Fat 2.9g (sat 0.4g)	Cholesterol 10mg
Protein 1.1g	Sodium 112mg
Carbohydrate 6.2g	Exchanges: ½ Starch, ½ Fat

Spoonbread

Yield: 6 (1-cup) servings

1½	cups boiling water
1	cup cornmeal
¾	teaspoon salt
2	tablespoons reduced-calorie margarine
1	cup fat-free milk
1	egg, separated
1	teaspoon baking powder
1	egg white
Cooking spray	

Pour boiling water over cornmeal gradually, stirring until smooth. Add salt and margarine, stirring until blended; cool 10 minutes. Stir in milk, egg yolk, and baking powder.

Beat egg whites at high speed of an electric mixer until stiff peaks form. Gently fold beaten egg whites into cornmeal mixture. Pour mixture into a 1½-quart baking dish coated with cooking spray.

Bake at 375° for 45 minutes or until lightly browned. Serve immediately.

Per Serving:

Calories 125	Fiber 2.2g
Fat 4.2g (sat 0.4g)	Cholesterol 38mg
Protein 4.7g	Sodium 378mg
Carbohydrate 18.0g	Exchanges: 1 Starch, 1 Fat

If you grew up eating spoonbread in your grandmother's kitchen, this lightened version should bring back some happy memories.

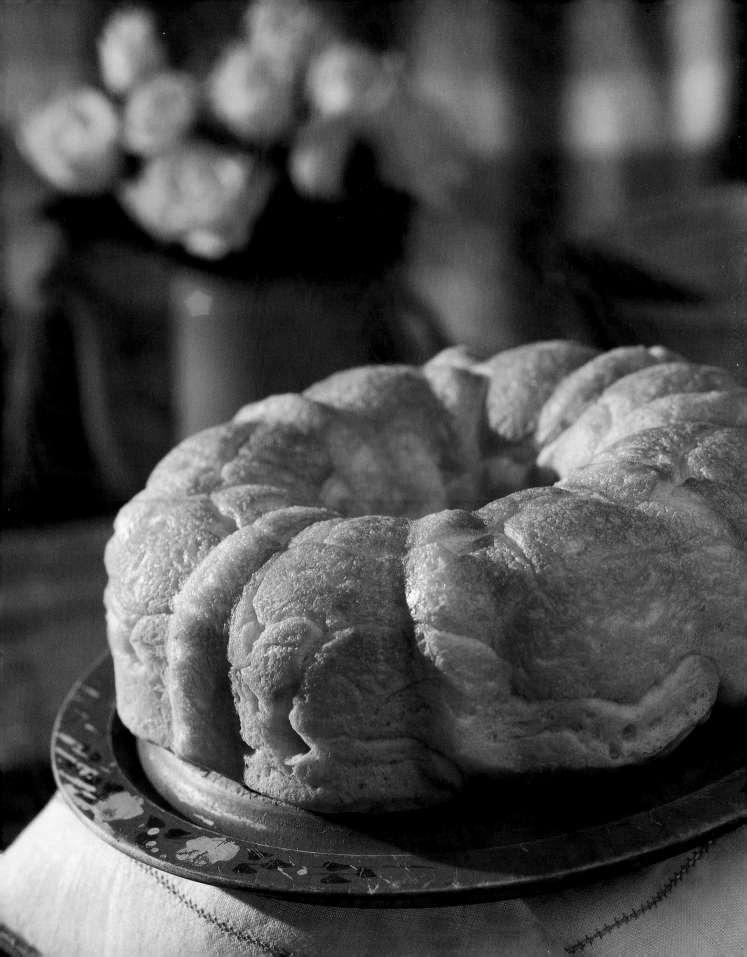

Monkey Bread

Yield: 18 servings (serving size: 2 balls)

1   package active dry yeast
1   cup warm water (105° to 115°), divided
2¾ cups all-purpose flour
2   tablespoons sugar
¾   teaspoon salt
3   tablespoons reduced-calorie margarine, melted
Butter-flavored cooking spray

Combine yeast and ¼ cup warm water in a 1-cup liquid measuring cup; let stand 5 minutes. Combine yeast mixture, remaining ¾ cup warm water, flour, sugar, and salt in a large bowl; beat at medium speed of an electric mixer until well blended. Cover and chill at least 8 hours.

Punch dough down. Turn out onto a heavily floured surface, and knead 3 or 4 times. Shape dough into 36 (1-inch) balls.

Brush balls with melted margarine, and layer in a 12-cup Bundt pan coated with cooking spray. Cover and let rise in a warm place (85°), free from drafts, 40 to 45 minutes or until doubled in bulk.

Bake at 350° for 30 to 35 minutes or until golden. Serve warm.

Per Serving:

Calories 86	Fiber 0.6g
Fat 1.5g (sat 0.0g)	Cholesterol 0mg
Protein 2.1g	Sodium 116mg
Carbohydrate 16.1g	Exchange: 1 Starch

Quick Yeast Rolls

Yield: 2 dozen

2 packages active dry yeast
½ cup warm water (105° to 115°)
1 cup fat-free milk
¼ cup fat-free egg substitute
2 tablespoons sugar
1 tablespoon vegetable oil
1½ teaspoons salt
4 cups all-purpose flour, divided
Butter-flavored cooking spray

Combine yeast and warm water in a 2-cup liquid measuring cup; let stand 5 minutes. Combine yeast mixture, milk, and next 4 ingredients in a large bowl. Gradually add 1 cup flour, stirring until smooth. Gradually stir in enough remaining flour to make a soft dough. Place in a bowl coated with cooking spray, turning to coat top, and let stand in a warm place (85°), free from drafts, 15 additional minutes.

Punch dough down; cover and let stand in a warm place (85°), free from drafts, 15 minutes.

Turn dough out onto a lightly floured surface; knead 3 or 4 times. Divide dough into 24 pieces; shape into balls. Place in 2 (9-inch) square pans or round pans coated with cooking spray, and let stand in a warm place (85°), free from drafts, 15 minutes.

Bake at 400° for 15 minutes or until golden. Serve warm.

Per Roll:

Calories 92	Fiber 0.7g
Fat 0.8g (sat 0.2g)	Cholesterol 0mg
Protein 3.0g	Sodium 156mg
Carbohydrate 17.7g	Exchange: 1 Starch

Desserts

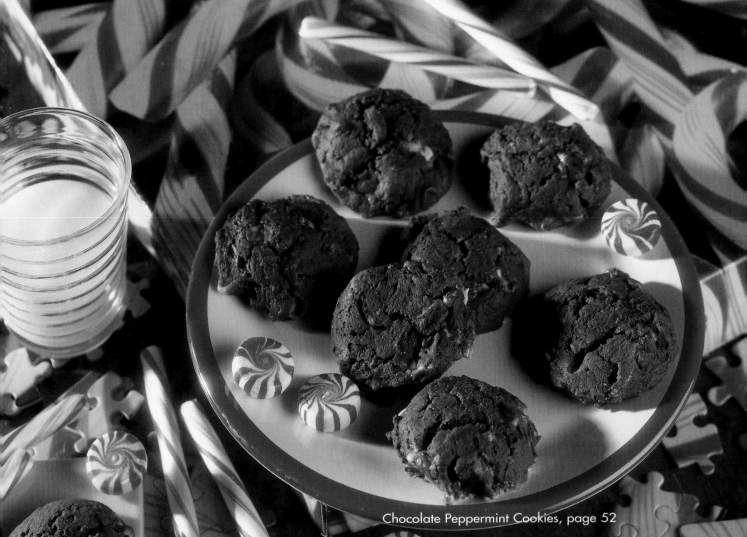

Chocolate Peppermint Cookies, page 52

Chocolate-Dipped Strawberries • Double-Chocolate Pudding Parfaits

Peanut Butter Ice Cream Sandwiches • Bananas Foster

Orange-Pumpkin Pie Desserts • Chocolate Chip Ice Cream

Chocolate Peppermint Cookies • Oven-Fried Peach Pies

Apple-Cinnamon Turnovers • Deep-Dish Cherry Pie

Raspberry-Mocha Cake • Banana Spice Cake • Mocha Angel Food Cake

Chocolate-Dipped Strawberries

Yield: 4 servings (serving size: 6 berries)

24   medium-size fresh strawberries
1   (2.8-ounce) sugar-free milk chocolate candy bar
1   tablespoon fat-free evaporated milk
2   teaspoons Grand Marnier or other orange-flavored liqueur
       (or orange juice)

Wash strawberries, and drain well. Do not remove caps.

Place chocolate in a small bowl. Microwave at HIGH 1 minute, stirring after 30 seconds. Stir until chocolate melts. Add milk and liqueur, stirring well with a wire whisk until smooth.

Insert wooden pick into center of each strawberry cap. Dip each strawberry halfway into chocolate mixture, and place on a baking sheet lined with wax paper. Refrigerate strawberries 30 minutes or until chocolate is firm. To serve, remove picks from strawberries.

Per Serving:

Calories 143	Fiber 2.9g
Fat 7.4g (sat 0.0g)	Cholesterol 5mg
Protein 2.4g	Sodium 21mg
Carbohydrate 20.0g	Exchanges: 1½ Fruit, 1½ Fat

Double-Chocolate Pudding Parfaits

Yield: 4 parfaits

1   (1-ounce) package white chocolate sugar-free,
        fat-free instant pudding mix
2   cups fat-free milk
4   sugar-free soft Rocky Road cookies, crumbled
        (such as Archway)

Prepare pudding mix according to package directions, using 2 cups fat-free milk; cover and chill.

Place 2 tablespoons crumbled cookies in each of 4 parfait glasses; top each with ½ cup pudding. Top evenly with remaining crumbled cookies, and serve.

Per Parfait:

Calories 168	Fiber 0.5g
Fat 5.2g (sat 0.2g)	Cholesterol 2mg
Protein 5.2g	Sodium 459mg
Carbohydrate 26.9g	Exchanges: 2 Starch, 1 Fat

Peanut Butter Ice Cream Sandwiches

Yield: 8 sandwiches

3   tablespoons no-sugar-added peanut butter (such as Smucker's
      Natural Creamy)
2   cups vanilla no-sugar-added fat-free ice cream, softened
16   (2-inch-diameter) gingersnaps

Swirl peanut butter into ice cream. Place in freezer 30 minutes or
until firm enough to spread.

Spread ¼ cup ice cream mixture onto each of 8 gingersnaps. Top
with remaining 8 gingersnaps. Place sandwiches on a 15- x 10-inch
jellyroll pan; freeze until firm. Wrap sandwiches in plastic wrap,
and store in freezer.

Per Sandwich:

Calories 124	**Fiber** 0.9g
Fat 4.7g (sat 0.9g)	**Cholesterol** 4mg
Protein 4.3g	**Sodium** 52mg
Carbohydrate 18.1g	**Exchanges:** 1 Starch, 1 Fat

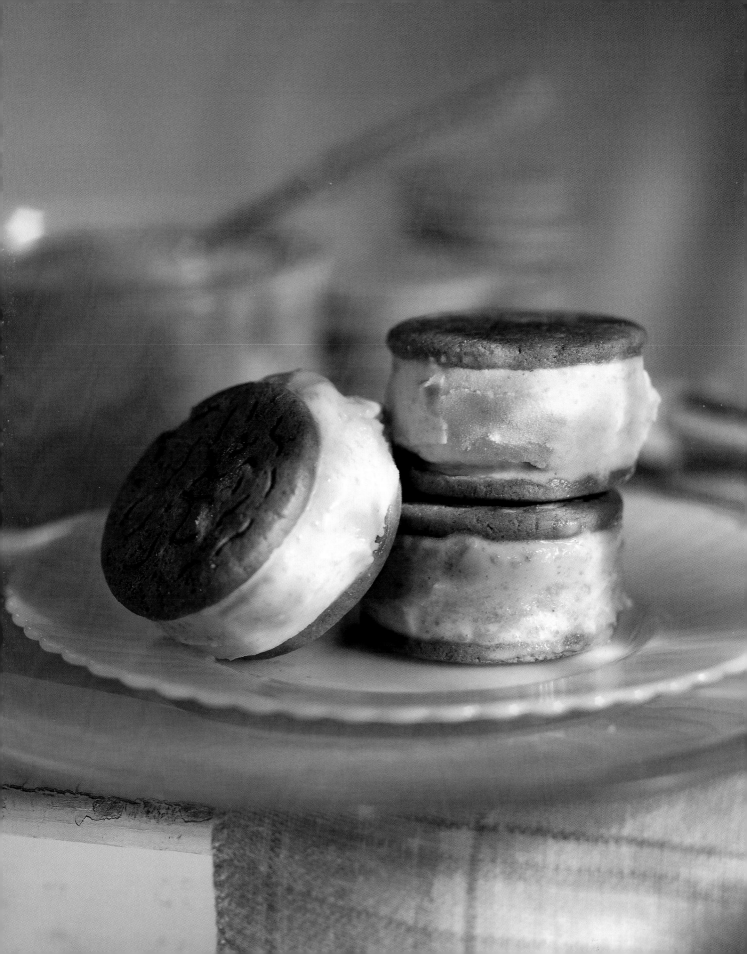

Bananas Foster

Yield: 6 servings

¾   cup unsweetened apple juice
⅛   teaspoon apple pie spice
3   medium-size ripe, firm bananas, peeled
2   teaspoons cornstarch
2   tablespoons rum
⅛   teaspoon maple flavoring
⅛   teaspoon butter flavoring
3   cups vanilla no-sugar-added, fat-free ice cream

Combine apple juice and apple pie spice in a large skillet. Cut bananas in half lengthwise; cut each half crosswise to make 12 pieces. Add banana pieces to juice mixture; cook over medium heat just until banana is heated, basting often with juice mixture.

Combine cornstarch, rum, and flavorings, stirring until smooth; add to banana mixture. Bring to a boil; boil, stirring constantly, 1 minute.

To serve, spoon ½ cup ice cream into each of six dishes. Spoon banana mixture evenly over ice cream, and serve immediately.

Per Serving:

Calories 164	Fiber 2.5g
Fat 0.3g (sat 0.1g)	Cholesterol 0mg
Protein 4.6g	Sodium 77mg
Carbohydrate 39.5g	Exchanges: 1½ Starch, 1 Fruit

Orange-Pumpkin Pie Desserts

Yield: 10 servings

½   cup canned mashed pumpkin
2   tablespoons orange juice
1   teaspoon pumpkin pie spice, divided
1½ cups vanilla no-sugar-added, fat-free ice cream, softened
½   cup orange sherbet, softened
2   tablespoons graham cracker crumbs (about 2 squares)

Combine pumpkin, orange juice, and ½ teaspoon pumpkin pie spice in a medium bowl; stir well. Add ice cream and sherbet, stirring well.

Spoon ¼ cup ice cream mixture into each of 10 paper-lined muffin cups. Combine graham cracker crumbs and remaining ½ teaspoon pumpkin pie spice. Sprinkle crumb mixture evenly over ice cream mixture. Cover and freeze until firm.

Serve in paper liners, if desired.

Per Serving:

Calories 53	**Fiber** 0.1g
Fat 0.3g (sat 0.1g)	**Cholesterol** 0mg
Protein 1.8g	**Sodium** 38mg
Carbohydrate 11.2g	**Exchange:** 1 Starch

This sweet and spicy dessert imparts all the flavors of rich pumpkin pie into an easy, make-ahead frozen treat—perfect for a holiday meal finale!

Chocolate Chip Ice Cream

Yield: 12 (½-cup) servings

⅔   cup granulated sugar substitute with aspartame
        (such as Equal Spoonful)
2   cups fat-free evaporated milk
1   cup fat-free milk
½   cup fat-free egg substitute
1½ teaspoons vanilla extract
2   (2.8-ounce) sugar-free milk chocolate bars, chopped

Combine first 5 ingredients in a large bowl; beat at medium speed of an electric mixer until well blended. Stir in chocolate.

Pour mixture into freezer can of 2-quart hand-turned or electric freezer. Freeze according to manufacturer's instructions. Let ripen for 1 hour, if desired.

Spoon into dessert dishes, and serve immediately.

Per Serving:

Calories 119	Fiber 0.0g
Fat 4.8g (sat 0.1g)	Cholesterol 5mg
Protein 6.0g	Sodium 88mg
Carbohydrate 14.3g	Exchanges: 1 Starch, 1 Fat

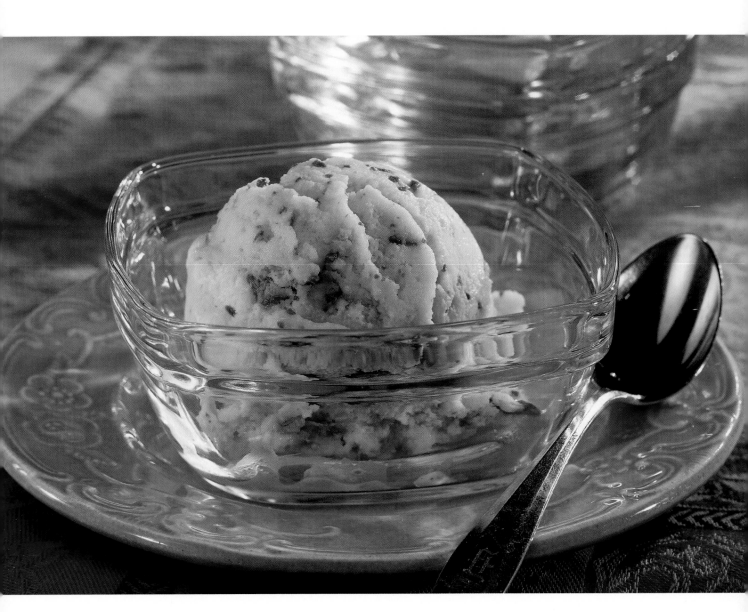

All I really need is love, but a little chocolate now and then doesn't hurt!

LUCY VAN PELT in Charles M. Schulz's "Peanuts"

Chocolate Peppermint Cookies

Yield: 38 cookies

½ cup margarine, softened
⅓ cup sugar
½ cup granulated brown sugar substitute (such as brown Sugar Twin)
½ cup fat-free egg substitute
1 teaspoon vanilla extract
2¼ cups all-purpose flour
1 teaspoon baking powder
¾ teaspoon baking soda
¼ teaspoon salt
⅓ cup unsweetened cocoa
⅔ cup finely crushed sugar-free peppermint candies (about 30 candies)
Cooking spray

Beat margarine at medium speed of an electric mixer until creamy; gradually add sugar and sugar substitute, beating well. Add egg substitute and vanilla; beat well.

Combine flour and next 4 ingredients. Add to margarine mixture, stirring just until blended. Stir in crushed candy. Drop dough by level tablespoonfuls onto wax paper. Roll into balls; place balls, 2 inches apart, on cookie sheets coated with cooking spray. Flatten balls with a fork. Bake at 350° for 10 to 12 minutes. Remove from cookie sheets, and let cool on wire racks.

Per Cookie:

Calories 70	Fiber 0.2g
Fat 2.7g (sat 0.5g)	Cholesterol 0mg
Protein 1.2g	Sodium 90mg
Carbohydrate 12.0g	Exchanges: 1 Starch, ½ Fat

(Photograph on page 43)

Oven-Fried Peach Pies

Yield: 10 pies

1	cup drained canned peaches in light syrup, chopped
3	tablespoons granulated sugar substitute (such as Sugar Twin), divided
¾	teaspoon ground cinnamon, divided
1	tablespoon all-purpose flour
1	(10-ounce) can refrigerated buttermilk biscuits

Butter-flavored cooking spray

Combine peaches, 2 tablespoons sugar substitute, and ½ teaspoon cinnamon. Sprinkle flour over work surface. Separate biscuits; place on floured surface. Roll each biscuit to a 4½-inch circle. Place 1 heaping tablespoon peach mixture over half of each circle. Brush edges of circles with water; fold in half. Seal edges by pressing with a fork.

Place pies on a large ungreased baking sheet; coat with cooking spray. Combine remaining 1 tablespoon sugar substitute and ¼ teaspoon cinnamon; sprinkle over pies. Bake at 375° for 10 minutes.

Serve immediately.

Per Pie:

Calories 116	Fiber 0.8g
Fat 4.3g (sat 1.0g)	Cholesterol 0mg
Protein 2.0g	Sodium 331mg
Carbohydrate 18.0g	Exchanges: 1 Starch, 1 Fat

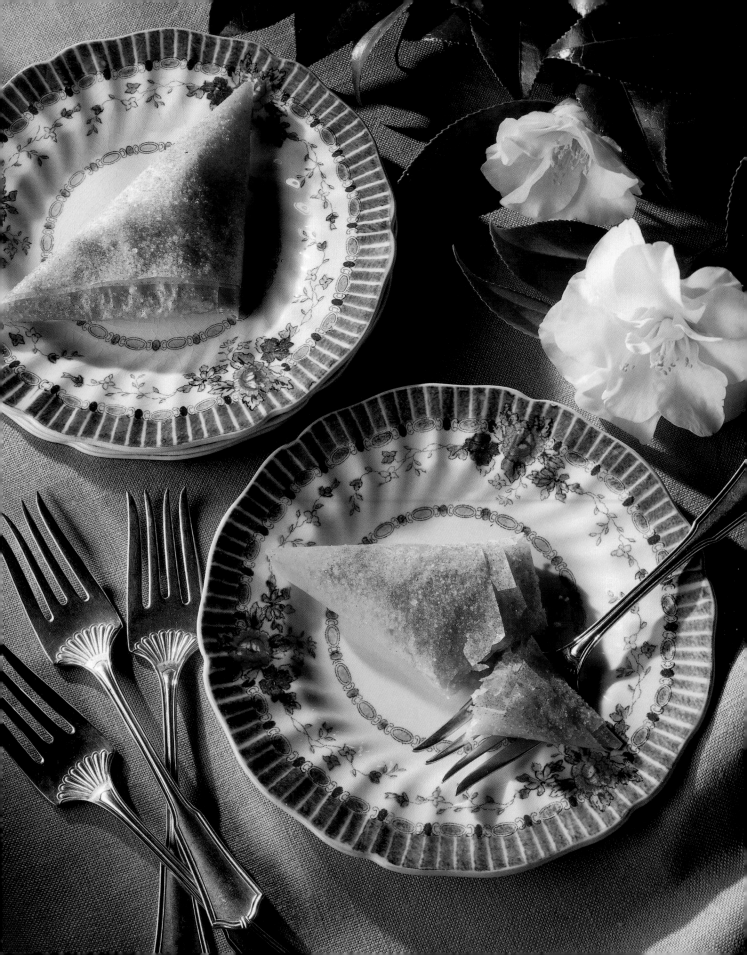

Apple-Cinnamon Turnovers

Yield: 8 turnovers

½ cup unsweetened applesauce
1 tablespoon currants
1 teaspoon all-purpose flour
¼ teaspoon ground cinnamon
⅛ teaspoon vanilla extract
4 sheets frozen phyllo pastry, thawed
Butter-flavored cooking spray
5 teaspoons granulated sugar substitute, divided
¼ teaspoon ground cinnamon

Combine first 5 ingredients; stir well. Place 1 sheet of phyllo on wax paper (keep remaining phyllo covered). Coat phyllo with cooking spray; sprinkle with 1 teaspoon sugar substitute. Top with 1 sheet of phyllo; coat with cooking spray, and sprinkle with 1 teaspoon sugar substitute. Cut stack of phyllo lengthwise into 4 equal strips, using a sharp knife. Repeat with remaining phyllo and 2 teaspoons sugar substitute.

Place 1 tablespoon applesauce mixture at base of 1 strip. Fold right bottom corner of phyllo over filling, making a triangle. Fold back and forth into a triangle to end of strip. Place, seam side down, on an ungreased baking sheet. Repeat with remaining phyllo strips and filling. (Keep covered before baking.)

Combine remaining sugar substitute and cinnamon. Coat triangles with cooking spray; sprinkle evenly with sugar substitute mixture. Bake at 375° for 10 minutes or until golden. Serve warm.

Per Turnover:

Calories 51	Fiber 0.3g
Fat 1.3g (sat 0.1g)	Cholesterol 0mg
Protein 0.8g	Sodium 49mg
Carbohydrate 8.9g	Exchange: ½ Starch

Deep-Dish Cherry Pie

Yield: 10 servings

1½ cups all-purpose flour
1½ tablespoons granulated sugar substitute (such as Sugar Twin)
¼ teaspoon salt
6 tablespoons vegetable shortening
6 tablespoons ice water
¾ teaspoon cider vinegar
4 (16-ounce) cans tart cherries in water
½ cup granulated sugar substitute
⅓ cup cornstarch
1 teaspoon ground cinnamon
½ teaspoon almond extract

Combine flour, 1½ tablespoons sugar substitute, and salt. Cut in shortening until mixture resembles small peas. Add ice water and vinegar; toss with a fork until moist. Shape into a ball. Roll into a 14-inch circle on a lightly floured surface. Place dough in a 10-inch pieplate; press against bottom and sides of plate. Flute edges.

Drain cherries, reserving 1¼ cups liquid. Set cherries aside. Combine reserved cherry liquid, ½ cup sugar substitute, and cornstarch in a saucepan; stir well. Cook over medium heat until very thick, stirring constantly. Stir in cherries, cinnamon, and almond extract.

Pour mixture into pastry shell. Shield pastry, and bake at 400° for 20 minutes. Reduce heat to 375°; bake, unshielded, 25 to 30 minutes or until hot and bubbly. Serve warm or at room temperature.

Per Serving:

Calories 220	Fiber 0.5g
Fat 8.0g (sat 2.0g)	Cholesterol 0mg
Protein 2.7g	Sodium 87mg
Carbohydrate 35.5g	Exchanges: 1 Starch, 1½ Fruit, 1½ Fat

Raspberry-Mocha Cake

Yield: 16 servings

2   (8-ounce) packages chocolate sugar-free, low-fat cake mix
1½ cups strongly brewed chocolate-almond flavored coffee
¼   cup raspberry spreadable fruit, melted
2   (0.53-ounce) packages sugar-free instant cocoa mix
1   (1.3-ounce) envelope sugar-free, reduced-calorie whipped topping
       mix (such as Dream Whip)
½   cup fat-free cold milk
½   teaspoon vanilla extract

Prepare cake mix according to package directions, substituting coffee for water. Pour batter into 2 (8-inch) round cake pans, following package directions. Bake at 375° for 20 to 25 minutes or until a wooden pick inserted into center comes out clean. Cool cakes in pans 10 minutes on a wire rack. Remove from pans. Poke several holes in each cake layer with a wooden pick. Brush warm cake layers with melted raspberry spread. Let cool completely on wire racks.

Combine cocoa mix and whipped topping mix in a large bowl. Add milk and vanilla; beat at low speed of an electric mixer until blended. Beat at high speed 4 minutes or until soft peaks form.

Place one cake layer on a serving plate; top with half of frosting. Top first layer with second cake layer; spread remaining frosting on sides and top of cake. Chill frosted cake until ready to serve.

Per Serving:

Calories 133

Fat 2.5g (sat 0.5g)

Protein 2.4g

Carbohydrate 28.1g

Fiber 0.7g

Cholesterol 0mg

Sodium 47mg

Exchanges: 2 Starch, ½ Fat

(Photograph on cover)

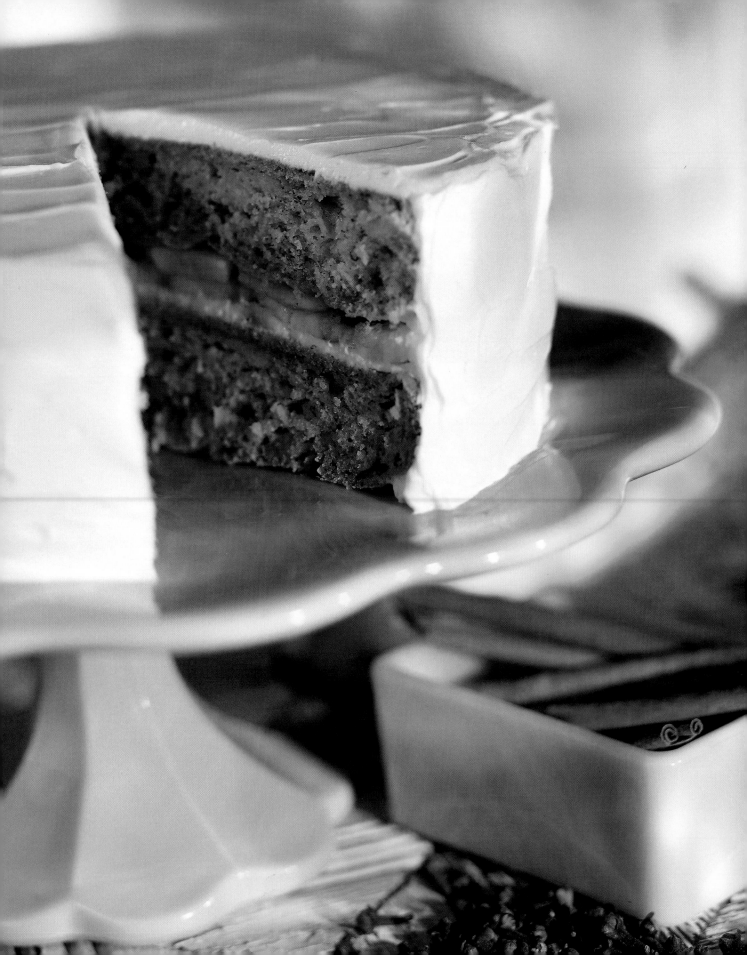

Banana Spice Cake

Yield: 16 servings

4   large ripe bananas, peeled and mashed (about 2 cups)
1½ cups vanilla nonfat yogurt sweetened with aspartame
¼   cup margarine, softened
2   eggs
2   teaspoons vanilla extract
3   cups all-purpose flour
1   tablespoon plus 1 teaspoon baking powder
2   teaspoons baking soda
½   teaspoon salt
1   teaspoon ground cinnamon
½   teaspoon ground cloves
1   cup granulated sugar substitute with aspartame (such as Equal Spoonful)
Cooking spray
2   (8-ounce) packages ⅓-less-fat cream cheese (Neufchâtel)
¾   cup granulated sugar substitute with aspartame
⅓   cup vanilla nonfat yogurt sweetened with aspartame
2   large ripe bananas, thinly sliced

Combine first 5 ingredients; beat at medium speed of mixer until blended. Combine flour and next 6 ingredients; add to banana mixture, beating well. Pour into 2 (9-inch) round cakepans coated with cooking spray and sprinkled with flour. Bake at 375° for 25 minutes. Cool in pans on wire racks 10 minutes. Remove; cool on wire racks. To prepare frosting, beat cream cheese, ¾ cup sugar substitute, and ⅓ cup yogurt just until smooth. Spread ½ cup frosting on one cake layer. Top with banana slices. Add second cake layer. Spread remaining frosting on top and sides of cake.

Per Serving:

Calories 235
Fat 9.4g (sat 4.5g)
Protein 6.6g
Carbohydrate 31.4g

Fiber 1.6g
Cholesterol 44mg
Sodium 465mg
Exchanges: 2 Starch, 2 Fat

Mocha Angel Food Cake

Yield: 12 servings

1¼ cups sifted cake flour
1 cup sugar, divided
⅓ cup unsweetened cocoa
1 teaspoon ground cinnamon
12 egg whites
1 teaspoon cream of tartar
1 tablespoon instant coffee granules
2 tablespoons warm water
1 teaspoon vanilla extract

Sift flour, ¾ cup sugar, cocoa, and cinnamon together three times.

Beat egg whites and cream of tartar in an extra-large bowl at high speed of an electric mixer until foamy. Gradually add remaining ¼ cup sugar, beating until soft peaks form. Sift flour mixture over egg white mixture, 1 tablespoon at a time; fold in gently after each addition. Combine coffee granules and water. Fold coffee mixture and vanilla into batter.

Spoon batter into an ungreased 10-inch tube pan; spread evenly with a spatula. Break large air pockets by cutting through batter with knife.

Bake at 300° for 50 minutes or until cake springs back when lightly touched. Remove cake from oven; invert pan, and cool completely. Loosen cake from sides of pan, using a narrow metal spatula; remove from pan.

Per Serving:

Calories 135	Fiber 0.3g
Fat 0.4g (sat 0.2g)	Cholesterol 0mg
Protein 5.1g	Sodium 54mg
Carbohydrate 27.5g	Exchanges: 2 Starch

Fish & Shellfish

Poached Salmon with Horseradish Sauce, page 69

Baked Striped Bass · Herbed Catfish Fillets · Peppered-Garlic Flounder
Greek-Style Flounder · Steamed Orange Roughy with Herbs
Poached Salmon with Horseradish Sauce · Creole Red Snapper
Grilled Trout · Lemon-Sauced Scallops · Spicy Shrimp Creole
Lemon-Garlic Shrimp · Barbecued Shrimp · Quick Paella

Baked Striped Bass

Yield: 4 servings

4   (4-ounce) striped bass steaks (¾ inch thick)
Cooking spray
2   tablespoons reduced-fat mayonnaise
1   teaspoon white wine Worcestershire sauce
½   teaspoon Old Bay seasoning
½   teaspoon lemon juice

Place fish in an 8-inch square baking dish coated with cooking spray. Combine mayonnaise and remaining 3 ingredients, stirring well. Brush mayonnaise mixture evenly over fish.

Bake, uncovered, at 450° for 8 to 10 minutes or until fish flakes easily when tested with a fork.

Transfer to serving platter, and serve immediately.

Per Serving:

Calories 147	Fiber 0.1g
Fat 6.2g (sat 1.2g)	Cholesterol 77mg
Protein 20.7g	Sodium 213mg
Carbohydrate 0.9g	Exchanges: 3 Lean Meat

Herbed Catfish Fillets

Yield: 4 servings

½ cup fine, dry breadcrumbs
¼ cup all-purpose flour
1 tablespoon chopped fresh parsley
1½ teaspoons chopped fresh dillweed
1½ teaspoons chopped fresh thyme
2 teaspoons chicken-flavored bouillon granules
1 teaspoon dried onion flakes
1 teaspoon paprika
¼ teaspoon garlic powder
4 (4-ounce) farm-raised catfish fillets
Butter-flavored cooking spray

Combine first 9 ingredients. Coat fish with cooking spray; dredge in breadcrumb mixture.

Place fish on rack of a broiler pan coated with cooking spray. Bake at 400° for 20 minutes or until fish flakes easily when tested with a fork.

Serve immediately.

Per Serving:

Calories 227	Fiber 1.0g
Fat 6.7g (sat 1.5g)	Cholesterol 66mg
Protein 23.6g	Sodium 635mg
Carbohydrate 17.0g	Exchanges: 1 Starch, 3 Lean Meat

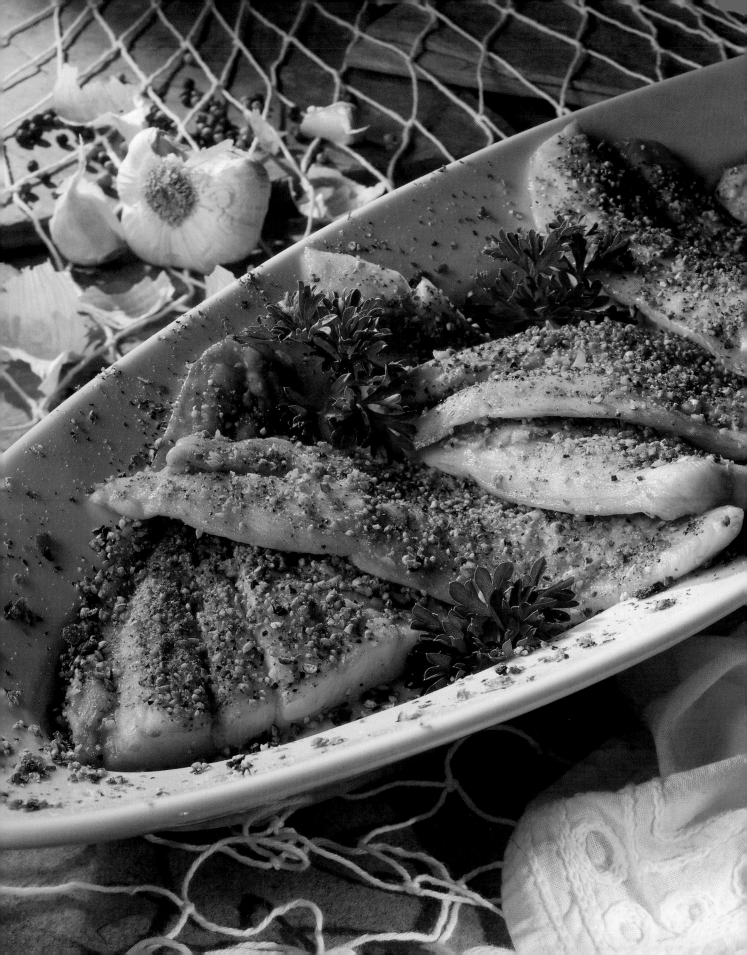

Peppered-Garlic Flounder

Yield: 6 servings

6 (4-ounce) flounder fillets
¼ cup low-sodium soy sauce
2 tablespoons minced garlic
1½ tablespoons lemon juice
2 teaspoons granulated sugar substitute (such as Sugar Twin)
1 tablespoon mixed peppercorns, crushed
Cooking spray
Fresh parsley sprigs (optional)

Place fish in a shallow baking dish. Combine soy sauce and next 3 ingredients; pour over fish. Cover and marinate in refrigerator 30 minutes.

Remove fish from marinade, and discard marinade. Sprinkle fish evenly with peppercorns, pressing firmly so peppercorns adhere to fish.

Place fish on rack of a broiler pan coated with cooking spray. Broil 5½ inches from heat 8 to 10 minutes or until fish flakes easily when tested with a fork.

Transfer to a serving platter, and garnish with parsley sprigs, if desired.

Per Serving:

Calories 113	**Fiber** 0.3g
Fat 1.5g (sat 0.3g)	**Cholesterol** 60mg
Protein 21.6g	**Sodium** 225mg
Carbohydrate 1.6g	**Exchanges:** 3 Very Lean Meat

Greek-Style Flounder

Yield: 4 servings

¼ cup lemon juice
1½ tablespoons balsamic vinegar
1 teaspoon dried oregano
1½ teaspoons olive oil
¼ teaspoon salt
⅛ teaspoon pepper
4 (4-ounce) flounder fillets
Cooking spray
3 tablespoons chopped fresh parsley

Combine first 6 ingredients in a small bowl.

Place fish in a 13- x 9-inch baking dish coated with cooking spray; pour lemon juice mixture over fish. Bake at 350° for 13 to 15 minutes or until fish flakes easily when tested with a fork.

Sprinkle with parsley, and serve immediately.

Per Serving:

Calories 115	**Fiber** 0.1g
Fat 2.4g (sat 0.4g)	**Cholesterol** 54mg
Protein 21.5g	**Sodium** 166mg
Carbohydrate 0.9g	**Exchanges:** 3 Very Lean Meat

Steamed Orange Roughy with Herbs

Yield: 4 servings

½   cup fresh parsley sprigs
½   cup fresh chive sprigs
½   cup fresh thyme sprigs
½   cup fresh rosemary sprigs
4   (4-ounce) orange roughy fillets
Lemon slices (optional)

Place a steamer basket over boiling water in Dutch oven. Place half of each herb in basket. Arrange fish over herbs in basket; top with remaining herbs.

Cover and steam 7 minutes or until fish flakes easily when tested with a fork. Remove and discard herbs.

Carefully transfer fish to a serving plate, and garnish with lemon slices, if desired.

Per Serving:

Calories 78	Fiber 0.0g
Fat 0.8g (sat 0.0g)	Cholesterol 23mg
Protein 16.7g	Sodium 71mg
Carbohydrate 0.0g	Exchanges: 2 Very Lean Meat

Use any combination of fresh herbs to infuse this fish with flavor.

Salmon are like men: too soft a life
is not good for them.

JAMES DE COQUET, French food writer

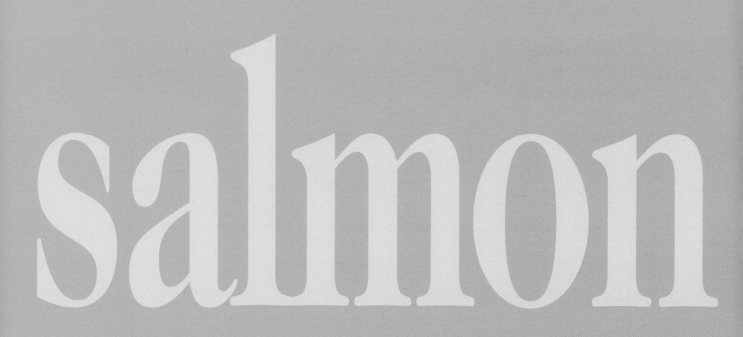

salmon

Poached Salmon with Horseradish Sauce

Yield: 4 servings

¼   cup nonfat mayonnaise
¼   cup plain nonfat yogurt
2   teaspoons prepared horseradish
1½ teaspoons chopped fresh or frozen chives
1½ teaspoons lemon juice
4   cups water
1   teaspoon peppercorns
1   lemon, sliced
1   carrot, sliced
1   stalk celery, sliced
4   (4-ounce) salmon fillets
Lemon wedges (optional)
Fresh celery leaves (optional)

Combine first 5 ingredients. Cover and chill.

Combine water and next 4 ingredients in a large skillet; bring to a boil over medium heat. Cover, reduce heat, and simmer 10 minutes. Add salmon to skillet; cover and simmer 10 minutes.

Remove skillet from heat; let stand, covered, 8 minutes. Remove fish from skillet. Discard liquid and vegetables.

Serve with horseradish mixture. If desired, garnish with lemon wedges and celery leaves.

Per Serving:

Calories 225	Fiber 0.0g
Fat 9.8g (sat 1.7g)	Cholesterol 77mg
Protein 25.1g	Sodium 452mg
Carbohydrate 7.5g	Exchanges: 1 Vegetable, 3 Lean Meat

(Photograph on page 61)

Creole Red Snapper

Yield: 4 servings

1	tablespoon olive oil
¼	cup chopped onion
¼	cup chopped green pepper
1	clove garlic, minced
1	(14½-ounce) can no-salt-added whole tomatoes, undrained and chopped
2	teaspoons low-sodium Worcestershire sauce
2	teaspoons red wine vinegar
½	teaspoon dried basil
¼	teaspoon salt
¼	teaspoon freshly ground pepper

Dash of hot sauce
4   (4-ounce) red snapper fillets
Fresh basil sprigs (optional)

Heat oil in a large nonstick skillet over medium-high heat until hot. Add onion, green pepper, and garlic; sauté until tender.

Add tomatoes and next 6 ingredients. Bring to a boil; add fillets, spooning tomato mixture over fish. Reduce heat; cover and simmer 12 minutes or until fish flakes easily when tested with a fork.

Garnish with basil sprigs, if desired, and serve immediately.

Per Serving:

Calories 173	Fiber 0.8g
Fat 5.0g (sat 0.8g)	Cholesterol 42mg
Protein 24.3g	Sodium 243mg
Carbohydrate 6.9g	Exchanges: 1 Vegetable, 3 Very Lean Meat, ½ Fat

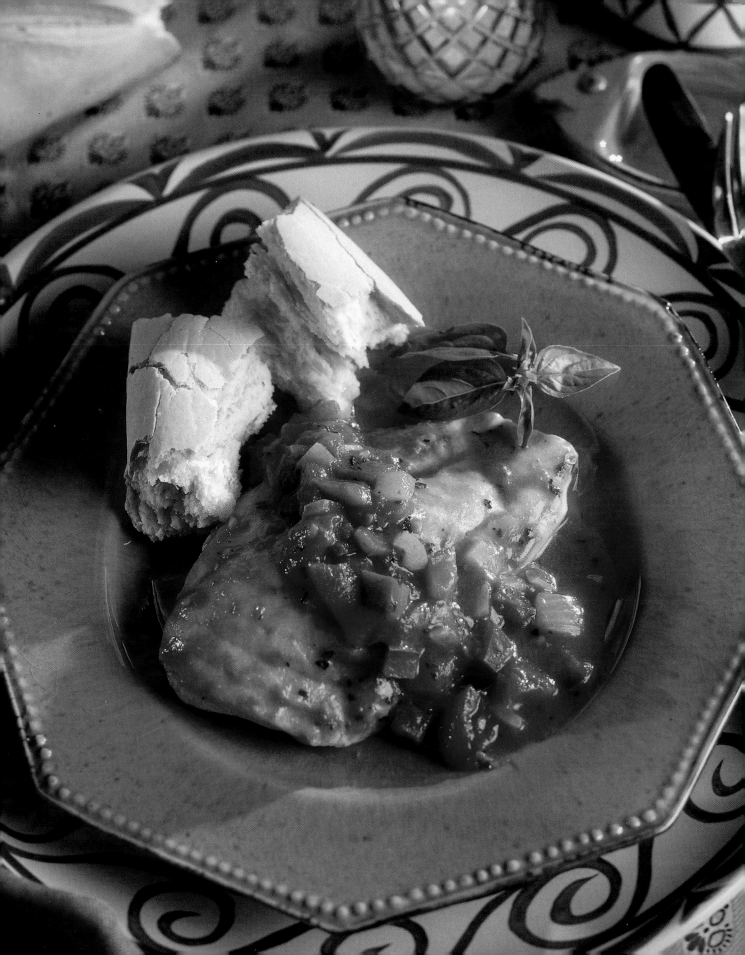

Grilled Trout

Yield: 6 servings

2   tablespoons herb-flavored or plain vegetable oil
¼   cup lemon juice
½   teaspoon salt
2   (2-pound) dressed trout
4   sprigs fresh tarragon
1   lemon, sliced
Cooking spray

Combine first 3 ingredients in a small bowl, stirring well with a wire whisk. Brush mixture inside each fish, using half of mixture. Place 2 sprigs tarragon and 2 lemon slices inside each fish.

Place fish in a 13- x 9-inch baking dish. Pour remaining oil mixture over fish. Cover and marinate in refrigerator 2 hours.

Place fish in a grill basket coated with cooking spray. Cook, covered, over hot coals (400° to 500°) 5 to 7 minutes on each side or until fish flakes easily when tested with a fork.

Serve immediately.

Per Serving:

Calories 206	**Fiber** 0.1g
Fat 11.8g (sat 2.1g)	**Cholesterol** 61mg
Protein 22.3g	**Sodium** 251mg
Carbohydrate 2.9g	**Exchanges:** 3 Lean Meat, ½ Fat

Substitute any fresh herb for the tarragon in this recipe.

Lemon-Sauced Scallops

Yield: 6 servings

¾ cup all-purpose flour
¼ teaspoon ground white pepper
1½ pounds fresh bay scallops
3 egg whites, lightly beaten
Cooking spray
1 tablespoon plus 1 teaspoon reduced-calorie margarine, divided
⅔ cup dry white wine or low-sodium chicken broth
½ cup sliced green onions
¼ cup lemon juice
⅛ teaspoon salt

Combine flour and pepper in a shallow dish; stir. Dip scallops in flour mixture; dip in egg white, and dip in flour mixture again.

Coat a nonstick skillet with cooking spray; add 2 teaspoons margarine. Place over medium-high heat until margarine melts. Add half of scallops; cook 6 minutes or until scallops are lightly browned, turning to brown all sides. Remove scallops from skillet; set aside, and keep warm. Repeat with remaining margarine and scallops. Add wine (or broth) and remaining 3 ingredients to skillet; cook 3 minutes or until mixture reduces to ⅓ cup.

To serve, arrange scallops on a serving platter; top with sauce.

Per Serving:

Calories 185
Fat 2.8g (sat 0.3g)
Protein 22.5g
Carbohydrate 16.5g

Fiber 0.6g
Cholesterol 37mg
Sodium 285mg
Exchanges: 1 Starch, 3 Very Lean Meat

Spicy Shrimp Creole

Yield: 5 servings (serving size: 1½ cups shrimp and ½ cup rice)

1   pound unpeeled medium-size fresh shrimp
Olive oil-flavored cooking spray
1   cup chopped onion (about 1 medium)
1   cup chopped green pepper (about 1 medium)
½   teaspoon dried crushed red pepper
6   cloves garlic, minced
2   (14½-ounce) cans Cajun-style stewed tomatoes, undrained
2½   cups cooked long-grain rice (cooked without salt or fat)

Peel and devein shrimp; set aside.

Coat a nonstick skillet with cooking spray; place over medium-high heat until hot. Add onion and next 3 ingredients; sauté until tender. Add tomatoes. Bring to a boil; reduce heat, and simmer, uncovered, 10 minutes, stirring occasionally. Add shrimp. Cover and cook 5 minutes or until shrimp turn pink.

To serve, spoon shrimp mixture over rice.

Per Serving:

Calories 247	Fiber 2.2g
Fat 1.6g (sat 0.3g)	Cholesterol 103mg
Protein 18.1g	Sodium 521mg
Carbohydrate 34.6g	Exchanges: 2 Starch, 1 Vegetable, 2 Very Lean Meat

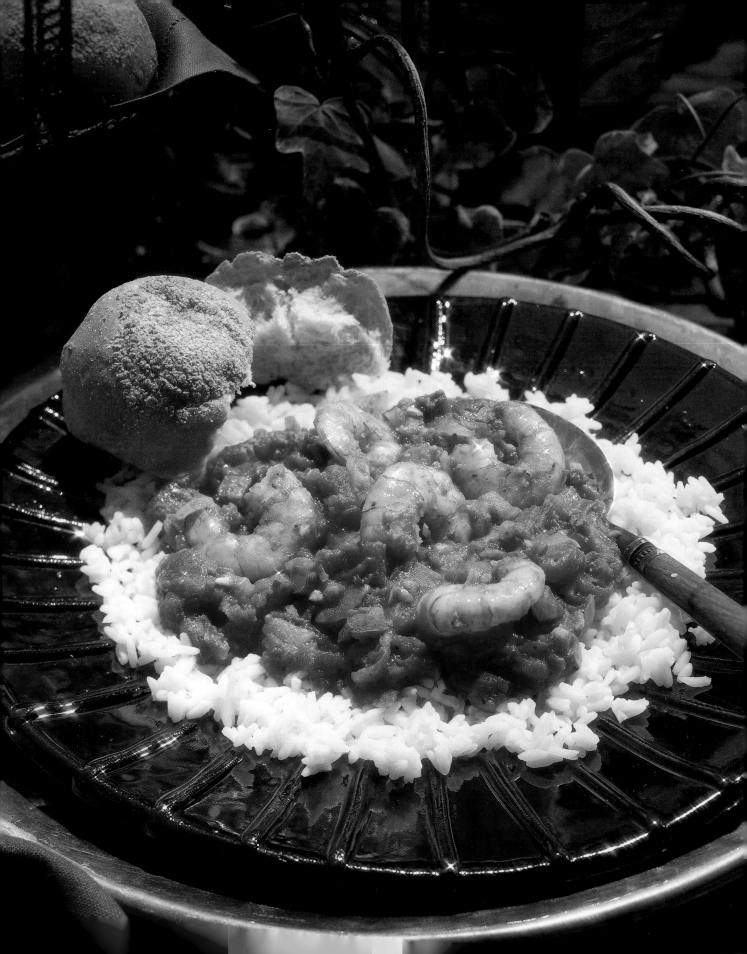

Lemon-Garlic Shrimp

Yield: 6 servings

2¼ pounds unpeeled jumbo fresh shrimp
Cooking spray
3 tablespoons minced onion
3 tablespoons minced fresh parsley
3 cloves garlic, minced
½ cup lemon juice
¼ cup fat-free Italian salad dressing
¼ cup water
¼ cup low-sodium soy sauce
½ teaspoon freshly ground pepper

Peel and devein shrimp, leaving tails intact. Place shrimp in a large shallow baking dish. Set aside.

Coat a nonstick skillet with cooking spray; place over medium-high heat until hot. Add onion, parsley, and garlic; sauté until tender. Stir in lemon juice and remaining 4 ingredients. Pour mixture over shrimp. Cover and marinate in refrigerator 1 to 2 hours, turning occasionally.

Uncover shrimp; broil 5½ inches from heat 5 minutes or until done, basting with marinade.

Serve with a slotted spoon.

Per Serving:

Calories 88	Fiber 0.2g
Fat 1.0g (sat 0.2g)	Cholesterol 157mg
Protein 17.1g	Sodium 289mg
Carbohydrate 1.7g	Exchanges: 2 Very Lean Meat

Barbecued Shrimp

Yield: 4 servings

24 unpeeled jumbo fresh shrimp, peeled and deveined
Cooking spray
¼ cup diced onion
½ cup reduced-calorie ketchup
2 tablespoons chopped fresh rosemary
1 tablespoon dry mustard
1 tablespoon granulated brown sugar substitute (such as brown Sugar Twin)
1 tablespoon white vinegar
¼ teaspoon garlic powder
Dash of hot sauce
1 lemon, cut into 4 wedges

Place shrimp in a large heavy-duty, zip-top plastic bag. Coat a nonstick skillet with cooking spray; place over medium-high heat until hot. Add onion; sauté until tender. Stir in ketchup and next 6 ingredients; pour over shrimp. Seal bag; shake until shrimp is coated. Marinate in refrigerator 1 hour, turning bag occasionally. Discard marinade.

Soak four 8-inch wooden skewers in water at least 30 minutes. Thread 6 shrimp onto each skewer.

Coat grill rack with cooking spray; place on grill over medium-hot coals (350° to 400°). Place skewers on rack; grill, covered, 3 to 4 minutes on each side or until shrimp turn pink. Squeeze 1 lemon wedge over each skewer, and serve immediately.

Per Serving:

Calories 145	Fiber 0.4g
Fat 2.0g (sat 0.4g)	Cholesterol 221mg
Protein 24.3g	Sodium 266mg
Carbohydrate 5.3g	Exchanges: 3 Very Lean Meat

Quick Paella

Yield: 6 servings

1	dozen fresh mussels
2½	cups canned low-sodium chicken broth
1	cup converted rice, uncooked
1	tablespoon curry powder
¼	teaspoon salt
1	cup frozen English peas
2	(8-ounce) packages chunk-style lobster-flavored seafood product
1	(7½-ounce) jar whole pimientos, drained and cut into 1-inch pieces

Remove beards on mussels, and scrub shells with a brush. Discard opened, cracked, or heavy mussels (they're filled with sand). Set aside.

Pour broth into a large saucepan, and bring to a boil; add rice, curry powder, and salt. Cover, reduce heat, and simmer 15 minutes. Add mussels, peas, seafood, and pimiento; cook 5 additional minutes or until mussels open and rice is tender. Discard unopened mussels.

Serve immediately.

Per Serving:

Calories 232	Fiber 1.7g
Fat 1.5g (sat 0.4g)	Cholesterol 8mg
Protein 13.2g	Sodium 697mg
Carbohydrate 40.4g	Exchanges: 2½ Starch, 1 Very Lean Meat

Use converted (parboiled) rice in this recipe so your rice won't be gummy.

Meatless Main Dishes

Vegetable Lasagna, page 90

Garden-Fresh Puffy Omelets

Yield: 2 omelets

½ cup fat-free egg substitute
2 tablespoons fat-free milk
1½ teaspoons minced fresh dillweed
¼ teaspoon salt
⅛ teaspoon pepper
4 egg whites
1 tablespoon all-purpose flour
Cooking spray
½ cup alfalfa sprouts
1 medium tomato, thinly sliced
1½ tablespoons freshly grated Parmesan cheese

Combine first 5 ingredients in a large bowl; set aside.

Beat egg whites at high speed of an electric mixer until soft peaks form; add flour, beating until stiff peaks form. Fold egg white into egg substitute mixture.

Coat a 6-inch nonstick skillet with cooking spray; place over medium heat until hot. Pour half of egg white mixture into skillet, spreading evenly. Cover and cook 5 minutes or until center is set. Layer half each of alfalfa sprouts, tomato, and cheese over half of omelet. Loosen omelet with spatula; fold in half. Slide omelet onto a plate. Repeat procedure with remaining egg white mixture, sprouts, tomato, and cheese. Serve immediately.

Per Omelet:

Calories 155	Fiber 1.7g
Fat 3.9g (sat 1.9g)	Cholesterol 8mg
Protein 19.0g	Sodium 677mg
Carbohydrate 11.1g	Exchanges: 2 Vegetable, 2 Lean Meat

Vegetable Burritos

Yield: 4 burritos

Cooking spray
1   teaspoon olive oil
2   cups sliced fresh mushrooms
½   cup chopped onion
½   cup chopped green pepper
1   clove garlic, minced
¾   cup drained canned kidney beans
1   tablespoon chopped ripe olives
⅛   teaspoon pepper
4   (8-inch) fat-free flour tortillas
¼   cup fat-free sour cream
¾   cup salsa, divided
½   cup (2 ounces) shredded reduced-fat sharp Cheddar cheese

Coat a large nonstick skillet with cooking spray; add oil. Place over medium-high heat until hot. Add mushrooms and next 3 ingredients; sauté until tender. Drain mixture, and return to skillet; stir in beans, olives, and pepper.

Spoon one-fourth of bean mixture down center of each tortilla. Top each with 1 tablespoon sour cream, 1 tablespoon salsa, and 2 tablespoons cheese; fold opposite sides over filling. Wipe skillet.

Coat skillet with cooking spray; place over medium-high heat until hot. Place burritos, seam sides down, in skillet; cook 1 minute on each side or until lightly browned. Serve with remaining salsa.

Per Burrito:

Calories 256	Fiber 3.4g
Fat 5.0g (sat 1.9g)	Cholesterol 10mg
Protein 12.9g	Sodium 648mg
Carbohydrate 40.4g	Exchanges: 2 Starch, 2 Vegetable, 1 Fat

Cheese and Onion Quesadillas

Yield: 4 quesadillas

Butter-flavored cooking spray
1   cup chopped onion (about 1 medium)
4   (8-inch) fat-free flour tortillas
1   cup (4 ounces) shredded reduced-fat sharp Cheddar cheese
½   teaspoon ground cumin
½   cup salsa
½   cup fat-free sour cream

Coat a large nonstick skillet with cooking spray; place over medium-high heat until hot. Add onion; sauté 5 minutes or until tender. Remove from skillet. Wipe skillet with a paper towel.

Coat skillet with cooking spray; place over medium heat until hot. Place one tortilla in skillet. Cook 1 minute or until bottom of tortilla is golden. Sprinkle one-fourth each of onion, cheese, and cumin over one side of tortilla. Fold tortilla in half. Cook tortilla 1 minute on each side or until golden and cheese melts. Repeat procedure with remaining tortillas, onion, cheese, and cumin.

To serve, top each quesadilla with 2 tablespoons salsa and 2 tablespoons sour cream.

Per Quesadilla:

Calories 237	**Fiber** 2.2g
Fat 5.8g (sat 3.2g)	**Cholesterol** 19mg
Protein 14.0g	**Sodium** 650mg
Carbohydrate 31.4g	**Exchanges:** 2 Starch, 1 Medium-Fat Meat

Spicy Vegetarian Tostadas

Yield: 6 tostadas

1   (16-ounce) can red beans, rinsed, drained, and divided
1   (15-ounce) can no-salt-added whole-kernel corn, drained
1   (14½-ounce) can whole tomatoes and green chiles
½   cup chopped green pepper
½   cup chopped onion
1½ teaspoons chili powder
6   (6-inch) corn tortillas
3   cups shredded lettuce
2   medium tomatoes, chopped
¾   cup (3 ounces) shredded reduced-fat sharp Cheddar cheese
¾   cup plain nonfat yogurt

Place 1 cup beans in a shallow bowl, and mash with a fork. Place in a medium saucepan; add remaining beans, corn, and next 4 ingredients. Bring to a boil; cover, reduce heat, and simmer 10 minutes. Uncover and cook until thickened and bubbly, stirring occasionally. Set aside, and keep warm.

Place tortillas in a single layer on a baking sheet; bake at 350° for 10 minutes or until crisp.

Spread bean mixture evenly on tortillas. Top with lettuce, chopped tomato, and cheese. Top each with 2 tablespoons yogurt.

Serve immediately.

Per Tostada:

Calories 271	Fiber 9.0g
Fat 4.0g (sat 2.0g)	Cholesterol 8mg
Protein 15.0g	Sodium 526mg
Carbohydrate 48.0g	Exchanges: 2½ Starch, 2 Vegetable, ½ High-Fat Meat

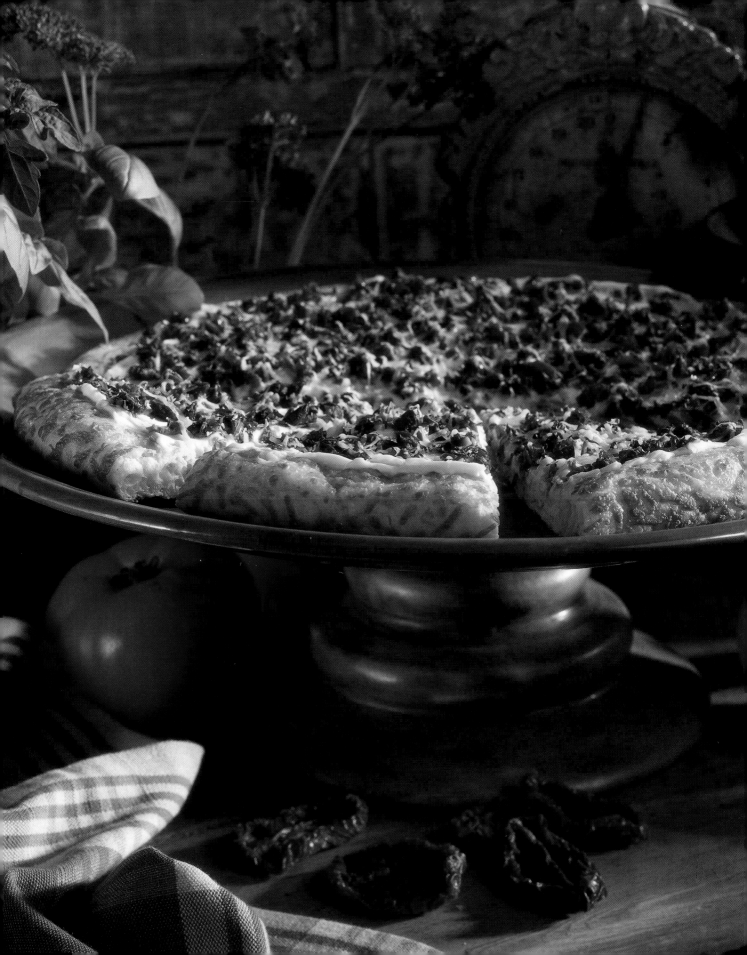

Ready in 30 Minutes!

Sun-Dried Tomato Pizza

Yield: 4 servings

12	sun-dried tomatoes (packed without oil)
¾	cup boiling water
3	cloves garlic
½	cup coarsely chopped fresh basil or parsley
⅛	teaspoon pepper
1	(10-ounce) thin-crust Italian bread shell (such as Boboli)
¾	cup ⅓-less-fat cream cheese (Neufchâtel), softened
3	tablespoons freshly grated Parmesan cheese

Combine tomatoes and boiling water; let stand 10 minutes. Drain. Position knife blade in food processor bowl. Drop garlic through food chute with processor running; process 3 seconds. Add basil and pepper; process until minced. Add tomatoes, one at a time, through food chute; process until minced.

Place bread shell on an ungreased baking sheet. Spread cream cheese over shell. Spoon tomato mixture over cream cheese, covering cheese completely. Bake at 450° for 5 minutes; sprinkle with Parmesan cheese. Bake 3 additional minutes or until cheese melts.

Per Serving:

Calories 310	Fiber 1.3g
Fat 12.7g (sat 6.2g)	Cholesterol 34mg
Protein 15.4g	Sodium 745mg
Carbohydrate 34.6g	Exchanges: 2 Starch, 1 Vegetable, 1 Medium-Fat Meat, 1 Fat

An unopened package of sun-dried tomatoes can be stored in the pantry up to one year; an opened package will keep for three months.

Thin-Crust Vegetable Pizza

Yield: 6 servings

1	(6½-ounce) package pizza crust mix
⅓	cup yellow cornmeal
⅔	cup hot water

Cooking spray

1	teaspoon vegetable oil
1	large onion, sliced
1	small yellow squash, sliced
1½	teaspoons salt-free herb-and-spice blend
¼	teaspoon salt
2	tablespoons fat-free Italian dressing
1	medium tomato, cut into 6 slices
1½	cups (6 ounces) shredded reduced-fat sharp Cheddar cheese

Combine pizza crust mix and cornmeal; add ⅔ cup water, stirring well. Shape dough into a ball; cover and let stand 5 minutes. Pat dough into a 14- x 11-inch rectangle on a large baking sheet coated with cooking spray. Bake at 450° for 5 minutes.

Coat a large nonstick skillet with cooking spray; add oil. Place over medium-high heat until hot. Add onion and squash; sauté 10 minutes or until vegetables are tender. Stir in herb blend and salt.

Brush crust with dressing; top with onion mixture and tomato slices. Sprinkle with cheese. Bake at 450° for 10 minutes or until crust is golden and cheese melts. Serve immediately.

Per Serving:

Calories 260	**Fiber** 2.6g
Fat 7.3g (sat 3.3g)	**Cholesterol** 19mg
Protein 13.4g	**Sodium** 529mg
Carbohydrate 14.2g	**Exchanges:** 1 Starch, 1½ Medium-Fat Meat

Pizza Pockets

Yield: 4 servings (serving size: 1 pocket plus ½ cup sauce)

Butter-flavored cooking spray
1   cup chopped zucchini (about 1 small)
½   cup chopped sweet red pepper (about ½ medium)
½   cup coarsely chopped fresh mushrooms
2½ cups pasta sauce, divided
1   (10-ounce) can refrigerated pizza crust dough
1   cup (4 ounces) shredded part-skim mozzarella cheese
2   tablespoons grated fat-free Parmesan cheese

**Making
Pizza Pockets**

Coat a large nonstick skillet with cooking spray; place over medium-high heat until hot. Add zucchini, red pepper, and mushrooms. Sauté 5 minutes. Stir in ½ cup pasta sauce; set aside.

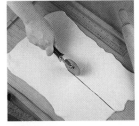

Step 1

Roll dough into a 15- x 10-inch rectangle; cut into 4 (7½- x 5-inch) rectangles (Step 1).

Spoon one-fourth of vegetable mixture onto one end of each rectangle (Step 2); sprinkle evenly with mozzarella cheese. Fold rectangles in half over filling; press edges together with a fork (Step 3).

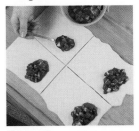

Step 2

Coat tops with cooking spray, and sprinkle with Parmesan cheese. Place on a large baking sheet coated with cooking spray. Bake at 400° for 12 minutes or until golden. Serve with remaining 2 cups warm sauce.

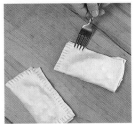

Step 3

Per Serving:

Calories 338	Fiber 3.9g
Fat 7.4g (sat 2.9g)	Cholesterol 16mg
Protein 16.0g	Sodium 840mg
Carbohydrate 50.0g	Exchanges: 3 Starch, 1 Vegetable, 1 High-Fat Meat

Potato-Vegetable Pie

Yield: 6 (1⅓-cup) servings

6   cups frozen mixed vegetables, thawed
1   (15-ounce) can kidney beans, drained
2   (8-ounce) cans no-salt-added tomato sauce
1   (4-ounce) can sliced mushrooms, drained
1   teaspoon chili powder
1   teaspoon low-sodium Worcestershire sauce
½   teaspoon salt
½   teaspoon pepper
Butter-flavored cooking spray
1⅓ cups fat-free milk
2⅔ cups frozen mashed potatoes, thawed
½   cup fat-free sour cream
¼   teaspoon salt
Paprika

Combine first 8 ingredients in a large bowl; stir well. Spoon mixture into an 11- x 7-inch baking dish coated with cooking spray.

Heat milk in a medium saucepan over medium heat until very hot. (Do not boil.) Stir in potatoes; cook, stirring constantly, 5 minutes or until thickened. Stir in sour cream and ¼ teaspoon salt. Spread potato mixture over vegetable mixture; sprinkle with paprika. Spray top with cooking spray. Bake at 350° for 40 minutes or until potato is lightly browned. Serve immediately.

Per Serving:

Calories 266	**Fiber** 7.9g
Fat 2.7g (sat 0.2g)	**Cholesterol** 3mg
Protein 13.5g	**Sodium** 641mg
Carbohydrate 48.0g	**Exchanges:** 3 Starch, 1 Vegetable, ½ Fat

In my family, mashed potatoes *are* the main dish.

CINDY PAWLCYN, American restaurateur and author

Potatoes

Squash Parmesan

Yield: 6 (1½-cup) servings

6   medium-size yellow squash
4   medium zucchini
2   eggs, lightly beaten
¼   cup water
⅔   cup fine, dry breadcrumbs
¾   cup grated Parmesan cheese, divided
⅓   cup minced fresh basil
¼   teaspoon dried crushed red pepper
3   cloves garlic, minced
2   teaspoons olive oil
Cooking spray
2   (15-ounce) cans no-salt-added crushed tomatoes, undrained

Cut each squash and zucchini lengthwise into 4 slices. Combine eggs and water, stirring well. Combine breadcrumbs, ½ cup cheese, basil, pepper, and garlic; stir. Brush vegetables with egg mixture. Dredge in breadcrumb mixture. Reserve remaining breadcrumb mixture.

Heat oil in a large nonstick skillet over medium-high heat. Add squash and zucchini to skillet; cook 3 minutes on each side or until lightly browned. Layer squash and zucchini in a 13- x 9-inch baking dish coated with cooking spray. Pour tomatoes over squash and zucchini. Top with remaining breadcrumb mixture. Cover; bake at 350° for 35 minutes. Uncover; sprinkle with cheese, and bake 25 minutes. Let stand 10 minutes.

Per Serving:

Calories 233	Fiber 3.2g
Fat 8.5g (sat 3.6g)	Cholesterol 86mg
Protein 13.6g	Sodium 389mg
Carbohydrate 28.1g	Exchanges: 1 Starch, 2 Vegetable, 1 High-Fat Meat

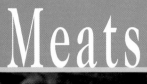
Meats

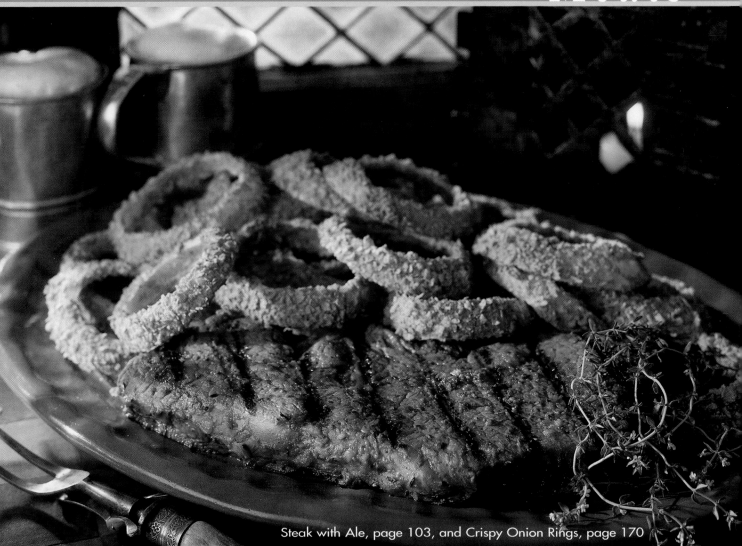

Steak with Ale, page 103, and Crispy Onion Rings, page 170

Lemon-Herb Cubed Steaks

Yield: 4 servings

1	cup fine, dry breadcrumbs
¼	cup grated Parmesan cheese
½	teaspoon dried Italian seasoning
¼	teaspoon salt
¼	teaspoon freshly ground pepper
3	egg whites, lightly beaten
1	teaspoon grated lemon rind
2	tablespoons fresh lemon juice
4	(4-ounce) cubed beef steaks

Olive oil-flavored cooking spray

Combine first 5 ingredients. Combine egg whites, rind, and juice. Dip steaks into egg white mixture; dredge in breadcrumb mixture.

Coat a nonstick skillet with cooking spray; place over medium heat. Add steaks; cook 8 minutes on each side or until tender.

Serve immediately.

Per Serving:

Calories 297	**Fiber** 1.2g
Fat 8.0g (sat 3.1g)	**Cholesterol** 65mg
Protein 32.8g	**Sodium** 578mg
Carbohydrate 21.5g	**Exchanges:** 1½ Starch, 4 Lean Meat

Cubed beef steak, taken from the top or bottom of the round, is not really cubed. Rather, it is tenderized by running it through the butcher's tenderizing machine.

Beefy-Tortilla Pie

Yield: 6 servings

Cooking spray
5   (6-inch) flour tortillas
½   pound ground round
1   (4.5-ounce) can chopped green chiles, drained
1   small onion, chopped
½   cup (2 ounces) shredded reduced-fat sharp Cheddar cheese
¾   cup fat-free egg substitute
½   cup fat-free milk
3   tablespoons all-purpose flour
½   teaspoon baking powder
½   teaspoon chili powder

Coat bottom and sides of a 9-inch pieplate with cooking spray and line with tortillas. Set aside.

Cook meat, chiles, and onion in a large nonstick skillet over medium heat until meat is browned, stirring until it crumbles. Drain. Add cheese; stir well. Spoon meat mixture into prepared dish.

Combine egg substitute and remaining 4 ingredients in a large bowl; beat with a wire whisk until well blended. Pour egg mixture over beef mixture. Bake at 350° for 45 minutes or until set. Serve warm.

Per Serving:

Calories 228
Fat 6.3g (sat 2.2g)
Protein 18.0g
Carbohydrate 24.1g

Fiber 1.8g
Cholesterol 30mg
Sodium 548mg
Exchanges: 1½ Starch, 2 Lean Meat

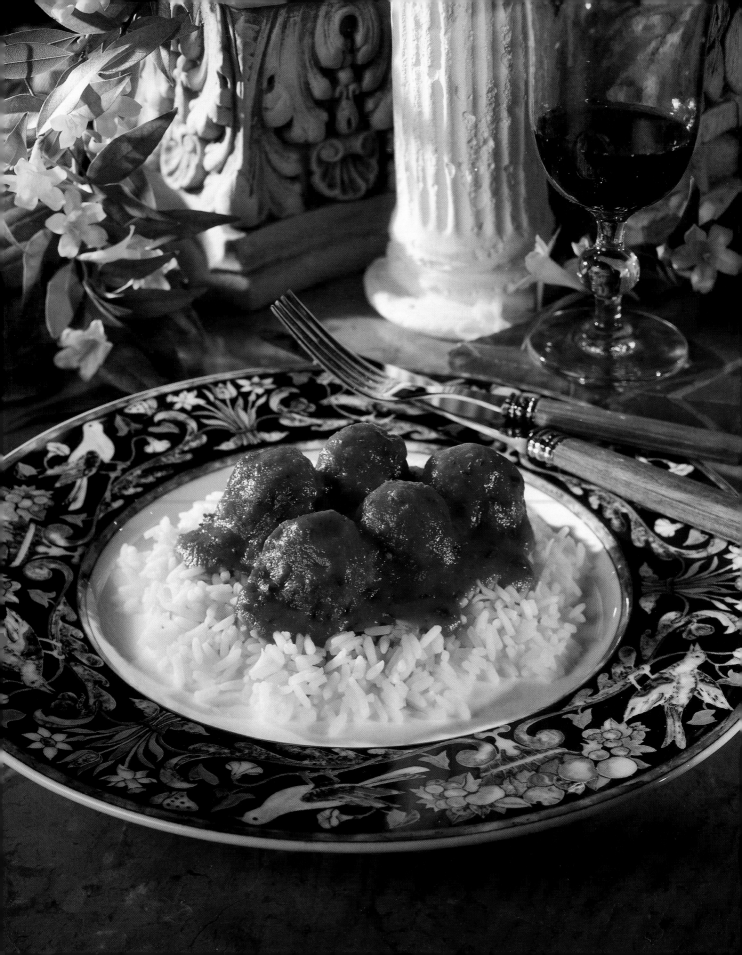

Greek Meatballs

Yield: 6 servings (serving size: 5 meatballs and ½ cup rice)

1   pound ground round
½   cup soft whole wheat breadcrumbs
2   tablespoons finely chopped onion
2   tablespoons fat-free milk
1   tablespoon chopped fresh parsley
1   teaspoon minced fresh mint
1   teaspoon Worcestershire sauce
¼   teaspoon salt
¼   teaspoon pepper
1   egg white
1   clove garlic, minced
Cooking spray
2   (8-ounce) cans no-salt-added tomato sauce
2   tablespoons chopped fresh parsley
1   teaspoon dried oregano
¼   teaspoon pepper
3   cups cooked instant rice (cooked without salt or fat)

Combine first 11 ingredients in a medium bowl; stir well. Shape into 30 (1¼-inch) meatballs. Place on rack of a broiler pan coated with cooking spray. Broil 5½ inches from heat 8 to 10 minutes or until browned, turning after 6 minutes.

Combine tomato sauce and next 3 ingredients in a large skillet; bring to a boil. Add meatballs; cover, reduce heat, and simmer 10 minutes or until thoroughly heated. Serve over rice.

Per Serving:

Calories 296	Fiber 0.9g
Fat 9.8g (sat 3.7g)	Cholesterol 47mg
Protein 19.3g	Sodium 202mg
Carbohydrate 32.3g	Exchanges: 2 Starch, 2 Medium-Fat Meat

Smothered Steak

Yield: 6 servings

1	(1½-pound) lean boneless round tip steak
3	tablespoons all-purpose flour
¼	teaspoon pepper
1	(14½-ounce) can no-salt-added stewed tomatoes, undrained
1	(10-ounce) package frozen chopped onion, celery, and pepper blend, thawed
3	tablespoons low-sodium Worcestershire sauce
1	tablespoon red wine vinegar
¼	teaspoon salt
3	cups cooked long grain rice (cooked without salt or fat)

Trim fat from steak; cut steak into 1½-inch pieces. Place steak in a 4-quart electric slow cooker. Add flour and pepper; toss. Add tomato and next 4 ingredients; stir well.

Cover and cook on HIGH 1 hour; reduce to LOW and cook 7 hours or until steak is tender, stirring once.

To serve, spoon evenly over ½-cup portions of rice.

Per Serving:

Calories 312	Fiber 0.6g
Fat 5.1g (sat 1.8g)	Cholesterol 68mg
Protein 27.9g	Sodium 225mg
Carbohydrate 36.5g	Exchanges: 2 Starch, 1 Vegetable, 3 Very Lean Meat

Using an electric slow cooker is like having a personal chef, but cheaper. Just throw some ingredients into the pot, go to work, and come home to a hot meal.

Simple Beef Stroganoff

Yield: 6 servings

¾   pound lean boneless top sirloin steak
Cooking spray
½   cup sliced onion
1   pound fresh mushrooms, sliced
¼   cup dry white wine or no-salt-added beef broth
¼   teaspoon salt
¼   teaspoon freshly ground pepper
1   (10¾-ounce) can reduced-fat, reduced-sodium cream of
         mushroom soup
½   cup fat-free sour cream
4½   cups cooked egg noodles (cooked without salt or fat)

Trim fat from steak; cut steak into thin slices. Coat a nonstick skillet with cooking spray; place over medium-high heat until hot.
Add steak; sauté 5 minutes. Add onion and mushrooms; sauté 5
minutes. Reduce heat to medium-low. Add wine, salt, and pepper;
cook 2 minutes.

Combine soup and sour cream; stir into steak mixture. Cook until
thoroughly heated. To serve, spoon meat mixture evenly over ¾-
cup portions of noodles.

Per Serving:

Calories 307	Fiber 4.1g
Fat 6.3g (sat 1.9g)	Cholesterol 78mg
Protein 21.7g	Sodium 357mg
Carbohydrate 40.2g	Exchanges: 2½ Starch, 2 Lean Meat

Cook the noodles while you're cooking the meat
mixture so that everything is ready at the same time.

Marinated Flank Steak

Yield: 4 servings

1   (1-pound) flank steak
2½ teaspoons prepared mustard
1½ tablespoons dry red wine
1½ tablespoons low-sodium soy sauce
1½ tablespoons lemon juice
1½ tablespoons low-sodium Worcestershire sauce
Cooking spray

Make shallow cuts in steak diagonally across grain at 1-inch intervals. Brush both sides of steak with mustard. Place steaks in a large shallow dish.

Combine wine and next 3 ingredients; pour over steak. Cover and marinate in refrigerator 8 to 12 hours, turning steak occasionally.

Remove steak from marinade, reserving marinade. Place reserved marinade in a small saucepan; bring to a boil. Remove from heat, and set aside.

Place steak on rack of a broiler pan coated with cooking spray. Broil 5½ inches from heat 5 to 7 minutes on each side or to desired doneness, basting with reserved marinade.

To serve, cut steak diagonally across grain into thin slices.

Per Serving:

Calories 226	Fiber 0.0g
Fat 13.2g (sat 5.6g)	Cholesterol 61mg
Protein 22.3g	Sodium 277mg
Carbohydrate 1.8g	Exchanges: 3 Medium-Fat Meat

Vegetables are interesting but lack a
sense of purpose when unaccompanied
by a good cut of meat.

FRAN LEBOWITZ, American humorist, *Metropolitan Life,* 1978

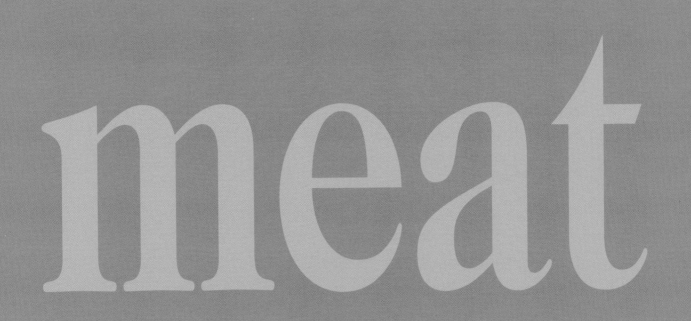

Grilled Sirloin with Red Pepper Puree

Yield: 4 servings

1	(1-pound) lean boneless beef sirloin steak (about ¾ inch thick)
¼	teaspoon salt
¼	teaspoon pepper

Cooking spray

1	(7-ounce) jar roasted red peppers, undrained
⅓	cup chopped green onions
2	tablespoons dry white wine or water
1	teaspoon beef-flavored bouillon granules

Trim excess fat from steak; sprinkle with salt and pepper.

Coat grill rack with cooking spray; place on grill over hot coals (400° to 500°). Place steak on rack; grill, uncovered, 8 minutes on each side or until desired degree of doneness. Set aside; keep warm.

Place peppers and liquid, green onions, wine, and bouillon granules in a skillet. Cover, reduce heat, and simmer 15 minutes. Cool sightly. Transfer pepper mixture to container of an electric blender; cover and process until pureed. Strain mixture, discarding liquid; return puree to skillet to heat thoroughly.

Cut steak into 4 equal portions, and place on a serving plate. Spoon one-fourth of red pepper puree over each portion. Serve immediately.

Per Serving:

Calories 186	Fiber 0.2g
Fat 6.5g (sat 2.5g)	Cholesterol 76mg
Protein 26.5g	Sodium 474mg
Carbohydrate 3.8g	Exchanges: 1 Vegetable, 3 Lean Meat

Steak with Ale

Yield: 6 servings

1	(1½-pound) lean boneless top sirloin steak, trimmed
½	cup finely chopped onion
½	cup boiling water
½	cup flat pale ale or light beer
1	tablespoon brown sugar
1	tablespoon red wine vinegar
1	teaspoon dried thyme
1	teaspoon beef-flavored bouillon granules

Cooking spray
Fresh thyme sprigs (optional)

Place steak in a shallow dish; set aside. Combine chopped onion and next 6 ingredients in container of an electric blender; cover and process until smooth. Reserve ½ cup ale mixture. Pour remaining ale mixture over steak; turn to coat. Cover and marinate in refrigerator at least 8 hours, turning occasionally.

Remove steak from marinade; discard marinade. Coat grill rack with cooking spray; place on grill over medium-hot coals (350° to 400°). Place steak on rack; grill, covered, 5 to 6 minutes on each side or to desired degree of doneness, basting frequently with reserved ½ cup ale mixture. Garnish with thyme, if desired.

Per Serving:

Calories 177	Fiber 0.2g
Fat 6.3g (sat 2.4g)	Cholesterol 76mg
Protein 26.0g	Sodium 110mg
Carbohydrate 2.3g	Exchanges: 4 Very Lean Meat

(Photograph on page 93)

Fruited Cider Roast

Yield: 12 servings

1   (3½-pound) lean boneless top round roast
¼   teaspoon salt
¼   teaspoon pepper
Cooking spray
6   cups unsweetened apple cider
3   cups cider vinegar
1   (6-ounce) package dried apricot halves, chopped
½   cup raisins
¼   cup granulated brown sugar substitute (such as brown Sugar Twin)
¼   teaspoon ground allspice

Trim fat from roast. Sprinkle roast with salt and pepper. Coat a large Dutch oven with cooking spray; place over medium-high heat until hot. Add roast, and cook until browned on all sides.

Combine cider and vinegar; pour over roast. Bring to a boil; cover, reduce heat, and simmer 3 to 3½ hours or until roast is tender. Transfer roast to a serving platter; set aside, and keep warm.

Skim fat from pan juices. Reserve 2 cups juices; discard remaining juices. Return 2 cups juices to Dutch oven; add apricots and remaining 3 ingredients. Cook over medium-high heat 10 minutes, stirring often. Serve fruit mixture with roast.

Per Serving:

Calories 239
Fat 5.6g (sat 1.9g)
Protein 28.4g
Carbohydrate 18.9g

Fiber 1.6g
Cholesterol 73mg
Sodium 111mg
Exchanges: 1 Fruit, 4 Very Lean Meat

Lemon-Pepper Veal Chops

Yield: 4 servings

⅓ cup lemon juice
2 tablespoons vegetable oil
⅛ teaspoon pepper
⅛ teaspoon hot sauce
4 (6-ounce) lean loin veal chops (¾ inch thick)
Cooking spray
Lemon slices (optional)

Combine first four ingredients, stirring well. Trim fat from chops; brush with lemon juice mixture. Set chops and remaining lemon juice mixture aside.

Coat grill rack with cooking spray; place on grill over medium-hot coals (350° to 400°). Place veal on rack; grill, uncovered, 4 minutes on each side or to desired degree of doneness, turning and basting frequently with reserved lemon juice mixture.

Transfer to a serving platter. Garnish with lemon slices, if desired.

Per Serving:

Calories 193	Fiber 0.0g
Fat 8.0g (sat 2.0g)	Cholesterol 100mg
Protein 27.2g	Sodium 77mg
Carbohydrate 1.8g	Exchanges: 4 Very Lean Meat, 1 Fat

Veal Cordon Bleu

Yield: 4 servings

8   veal cutlets (about 1 pound)
½   teaspoon freshly ground pepper
2   (¾-ounce) slices fat-free Swiss cheese
1   (1-ounce) slice lean cooked ham
2   tablespoons all-purpose flour
¼   cup plus 2 tablespoons fat-free egg substitute
½   cup fine, dry breadcrumbs
Cooking spray
1   tablespoon reduced-calorie margarine
Fresh parsley sprigs (optional)
Lemon slices (optional)

Place cutlets between 2 sheets of wax paper, and flatten to ⅛-inch thickness. Sprinkle 4 cutlets with pepper. Cut each cheese slice in half; place 1 half-slice in center of each of 4 peppered cutlets. Cut ham slice into 4 pieces; place evenly on top of cheese. Place remaining 4 cutlets over ham; pound edges to seal.

Dredge cutlets in flour. Dip in egg substitute; dredge in breadcrumbs. Coat a large nonstick skillet with cooking spray; add margarine. Place over medium-high heat until margarine melts. Add cutlets; cook 2 minutes on each side or until lightly browned. Place in an 11- x 7-inch baking dish coated with cooking spray. Bake, uncovered, at 375° for 20 minutes. Garnish with parsley sprigs and lemon slices.

Per Serving:

Calories 245	Fiber 0.5g
Fat 7.0g (sat 1.9g)	Cholesterol 98mg
Protein 31.1g	Sodium 489mg
Carbohydrate 12.7g	Exchanges: 1 Starch, 4 Lean Meat

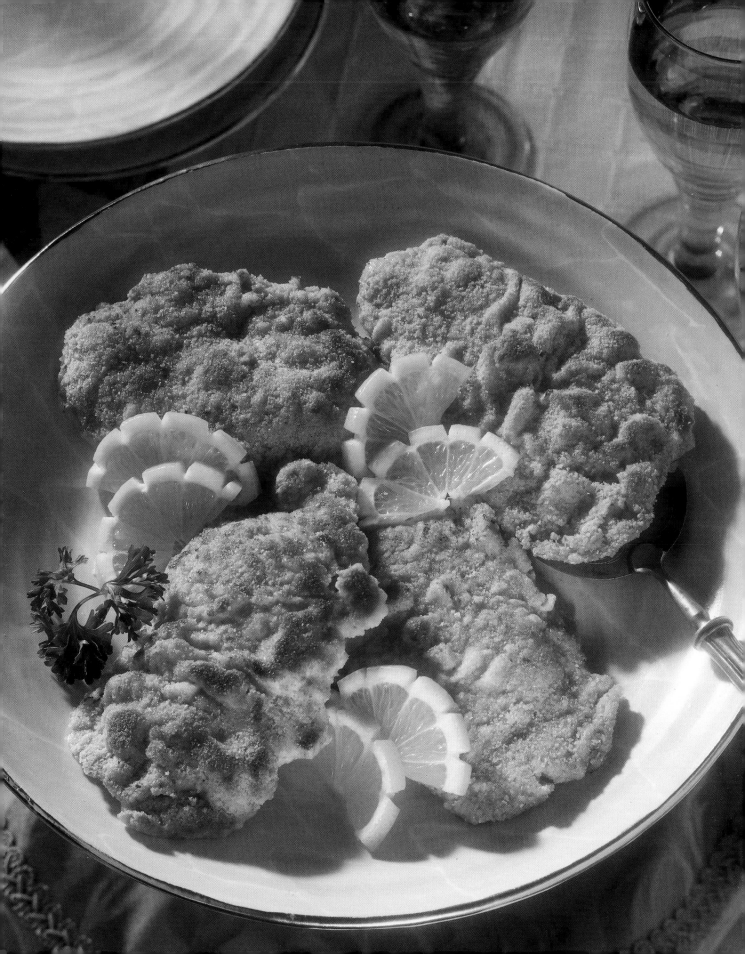

Lamb Shish Kabobs

Yield: 4 servings (serving size: 2 skewers)

1   pound lean boneless lamb
⅓   cup lime juice
1   tablespoon grated onion
1½   teaspoons chili powder
1   teaspoon ground ginger
1   teaspoon ground turmeric
1   teaspoon minced garlic
2   tablespoons water
1½   teaspoons olive oil
2   medium onions
1   large green pepper, cut into 1-inch pieces
16   medium-size fresh mushrooms
Cooking spray

Trim fat from lamb; cut lamb into 1¼-inch cubes. Place in a shallow dish. Combine lime juice and next 7 ingredients; pour over lamb. Cover and marinate in refrigerator at least 4 hours.

Cook 2 onions in boiling water to cover in a saucepan 10 minutes. Drain; cut each onion into 4 wedges. Remove lamb from marinade, reserving marinade. Place marinade in a saucepan, and bring to a boil. Remove from heat. Thread lamb, onion, green pepper, and mushrooms onto 8 (10-inch) skewers. Coat grill rack with cooking spray; place on grill over medium-hot coals (350° to 400°). Place kabobs on rack; grill, covered, 13 to 15 minutes or until lamb is done, turning and basting frequently with reserved marinade.

Per Serving:

Calories 254	Fiber 3.6g
Fat 9.3g (sat 2.7g)	Cholesterol 76mg
Protein 27.1g	Sodium 75mg
Carbohydrate 16.5g	Exchanges: 3 Vegetable, 3 Lean Meat

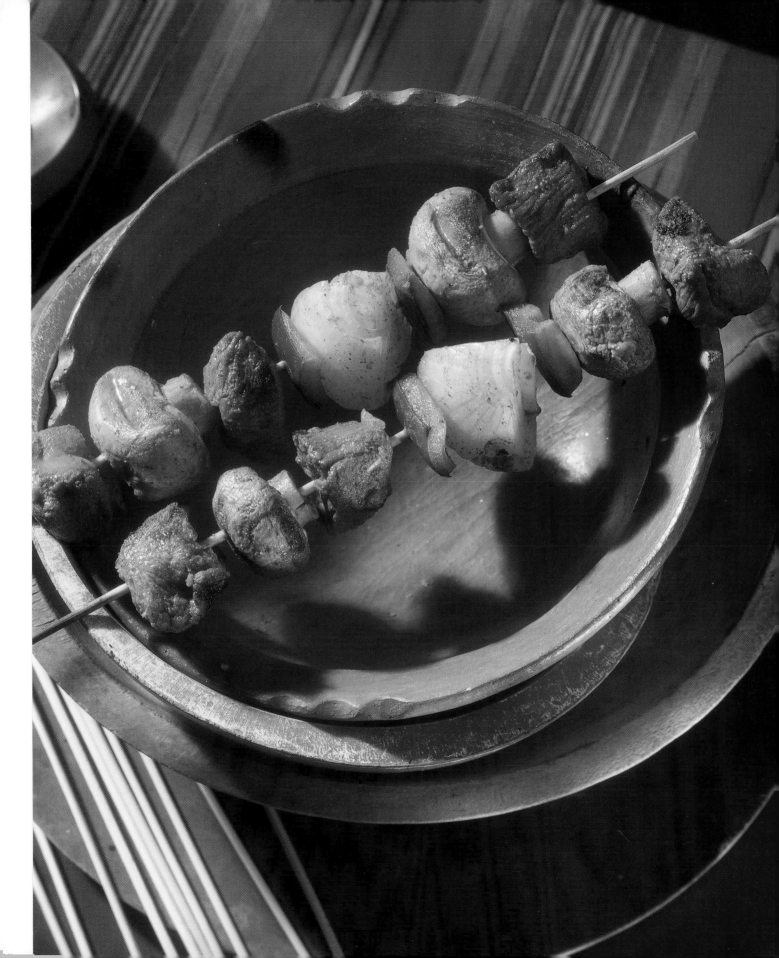

Pork Marsala

Yield: 4 servings

1	(1-pound) pork tenderloin
¼	cup all-purpose flour
⅛	teaspoon salt
1	tablespoon margarine
¾	cup Marsala wine
1	teaspoon beef-flavored bouillon granules
¼	teaspoon freshly ground pepper
3	cups cooked capellini (cooked without salt or fat)

Trim fat from tenderloin; cut tenderloin into ½-inch-thick slices. Combine flour and salt in a heavy-duty, zip-top plastic bag. Add tenderloin; seal bag, and shake until tenderloin is well coated.

Melt margarine in a nonstick skillet over medium heat. Add tenderloin; cook until browned, turning once. Remove from skillet. Add wine, bouillon granules, and pepper to skillet; bring to a boil. Reduce heat, and simmer, uncovered, 2 minutes. Return tenderloin to skillet; cover and simmer 2 minutes or until sauce is thickened.

To serve, spoon pork mixture evenly over ¾-cup portions of pasta.

Per Serving:

Calories 340	Fiber 1.9g
Fat 6.6g (sat 1.7g)	Cholesterol 74mg
Protein 29.7g	Sodium 403mg
Carbohydrate 37.6g	Exchanges: 2½ Starch, 3 Lean Meat

Indonesian Pork Tenderloin

Yield: 4 servings

1	(1-pound) pork tenderloin
2	tablespoons low-sodium soy sauce
2	tablespoons reduced-fat creamy peanut butter
1	teaspoon dried crushed red pepper
2	cloves garlic, minced
Cooking spray	
¼	cup apricot spreadable fruit

Trim fat from tenderloin. Combine soy sauce and next 3 ingredients, stirring well. Spread soy sauce mixture over tenderloin.

Place on a rack in a roasting pan coated with cooking spray. Insert meat thermometer into thickest part of tenderloin, if desired. Bake uncovered, at 375° for 30 minutes. Brush tenderloin with apricot spread. Bake 10 additional minutes or until meat thermometer registers 160°, basting often with apricot spread. Let stand 10 minutes before slicing.

Per Serving:

Calories 222	Fiber 0.5g
Fat 8.3g (sat 2.3g)	Cholesterol 79mg
Protein 26.6g	Sodium 285mg
Carbohydrate 8.0g	Exchanges: ½ Starch, 3 Lean Meat

Nothing helps scenery like ham and eggs.

MARK TWAIN

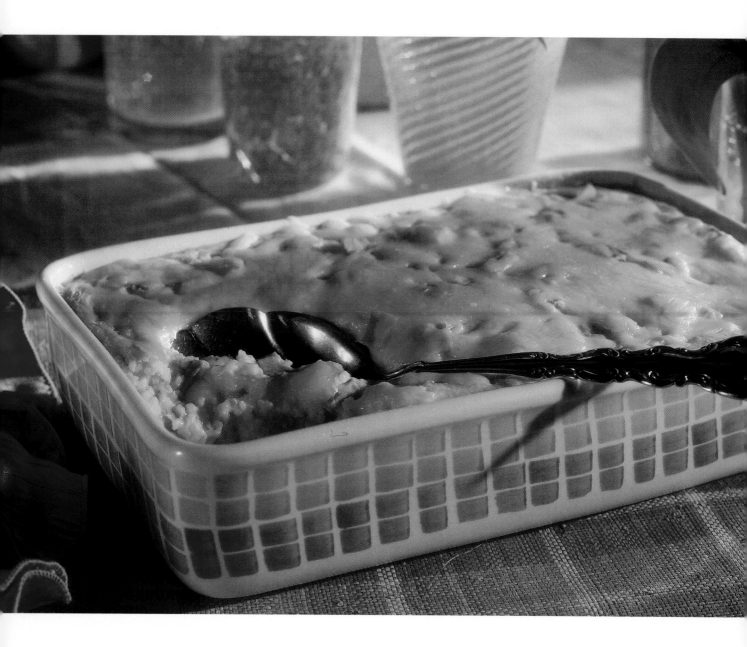

Ham and Grits Casserole

Yield: 6 (1-cup) servings

4   cups water
¼   teaspoon salt
1   cup quick-cooking grits, uncooked
1   cup chopped reduced-fat, low-salt ham
3   tablespoons reduced-calorie margarine
1   teaspoon low-sodium Worcestershire sauce
1   cup fat-free egg substitute
Cooking spray
½   cup (2 ounces) shredded reduced-fat sharp Cheddar cheese

Combine 4 cups water and salt in a large saucepan; bring to a boil. Stir in grits; cover, reduce heat, and simmer 5 minutes or until grits are thickened, stirring occasionally. Remove from heat. Add ham, margarine, and Worcestershire sauce; stir until margarine melts. Gradually add egg substitute, stirring well.

Spoon grits mixture into a 11- x 7-inch baking dish coated with cooking spray. Bake at 350° for 45 minutes. Sprinkle with cheese. Bake 5 additional minutes or until cheese melts. Let stand 5 minutes before serving.

Per Serving:

Calories 221	Fiber 1.5g
Fat 7.1g (sat 2.4g)	Cholesterol 19mg
Protein 14.1g	Sodium 487mg
Carbohydrate 26.0g	Exchanges: 2 Starch, 1 Medium-Fat Meat

Red Beans and Rice

Yield: 8 servings

Cooking spray
6 ounces low-fat smoked sausage, thinly sliced
1 cup chopped onion
¾ cup chopped green pepper
1 clove garlic, minced
3 (16-ounce) cans red beans, drained
1 (14½-ounce) can no-salt-added stewed tomatoes, undrained and chopped
1½ cups water
1 (6-ounce) can no-salt-added tomato paste
¼ teaspoon dried oregano
¼ teaspoon dried thyme
¼ teaspoon hot sauce
1 bay leaf
4 cups cooked long-grain rice (cooked without salt or fat)

Coat a Dutch oven with cooking spray. Place over medium-high heat until hot. Add sausage and next 3 ingredients; sauté until tender.

Add beans and next 7 ingredients; bring to a boil. Cover, reduce heat, and simmer 20 minutes or until thoroughly heated. Remove and discard bay leaf. To serve, spoon bean mixture evenly over ½-cup portions of rice.

Per Serving:

Calories 310	Fiber 5.7g
Fat 1.2g (sat 0.3g)	Cholesterol 9mg
Protein 15.9g	Sodium 448mg
Carbohydrate 59.2g	Exchanges: 4 Starch, ½ Lean Meat

Poultry

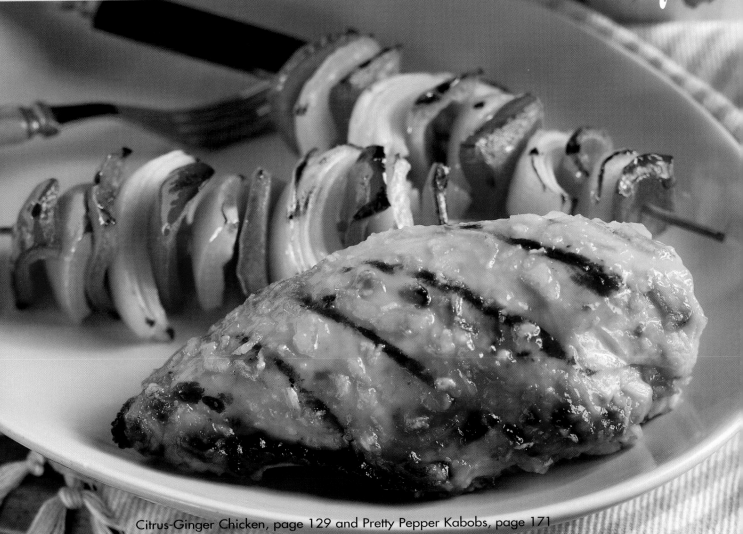

Citrus-Ginger Chicken, page 129 and Pretty Pepper Kabobs, page 171

Chicken Casserole

Yield: 8 (1-cup) servings

6	(6-ounce) skinned chicken breast halves
4	cups water
1	teaspoon pepper
1	(10¾-ounce) can reduced-fat cream of chicken soup, undiluted
1	(10¾-ounce) can reduced-fat cream of celery soup, undiluted
1	(8-ounce) carton reduced-fat sour cream
½	teaspoon pepper
8	ounces reduced-fat oval-shaped buttery crackers, crushed (about 80 crackers)
	Cooking spray
2	tablespoons margarine, melted

Combine first 3 ingredients in a large Dutch oven; bring to a boil. Cover, reduce heat, and simmer 1 hour or until tender. Remove chicken, and cool slightly.

Bone chicken; cut chicken into bite-size pieces. Combine chicken, chicken soup, and next 3 ingredients, stirring well.

Place half of crushed crackers in an 11- x 7-inch baking dish coated with cooking spray; spoon chicken mixture evenly over crackers. Top with remaining crackers, and drizzle with margarine.

Bake, uncovered, at 325° for 35 minutes or until lightly browned.

Per Serving:

Calories 306	Fiber 0.1g
Fat 12.9g (sat 4.4g)	Cholesterol 79mg
Protein 26.3g	Sodium 543mg
Carbohydrate 17.0g	Exchanges: 1 Starch, 3 Lean Meat, 1 Fat

Salsa Chicken

Yield: 4 servings

6   (6-inch) corn tortillas
Cooking spray
2   cups chopped cooked chicken breast
½   cup salsa, divided
2   cups chopped onion (about 2 medium)
1   (4½-ounce) can chopped green chiles, undrained
1   cup (4 ounces) shredded reduced-fat Monterey Jack cheese
½   cup fat-free sour cream, divided

Cut tortillas into ½-inch-wide strips (see photo). Place strips in a single layer on an ungreased baking sheet, and coat strips with cooking spray. Bake at 350° for 10 minutes or until crisp. Let cool.

Combine chicken and ¼ cup salsa in a large nonstick skillet. Bring to a boil over high heat. Reduce heat to medium-high, and cook 2 minutes, stirring occasionally. Remove from skillet; wipe skillet.

Coat skillet with cooking spray; place over medium-high heat until hot. Add onion; sauté 2 minutes. Add green chiles; sauté 2 minutes. Add cheese and ¼ cup sour cream; stir until cheese melts.

To serve, arrange tortilla strips evenly on serving plates. Top strips evenly with chicken mixture. Spoon onion mixture evenly over chicken mixture. Top each serving with 1 tablespoon salsa and 1 tablespoon sour cream.

Cutting Tortillas

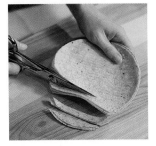

Per Serving:

Calories 333	Fiber 3.2g
Fat 9.2g (sat 4.0g)	Cholesterol 79mg
Protein 35.1g	Sodium 531mg
Carbohydrate 25.7g	Exchanges: 1½ Starch, 1 Vegetable, 4 Lean Meat

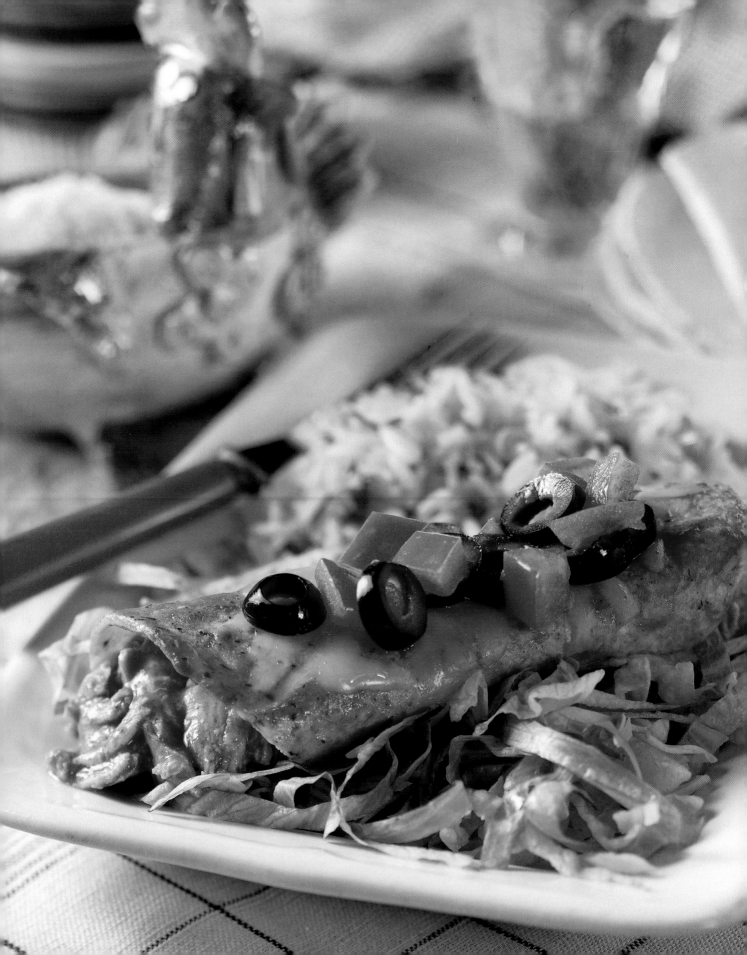

Chicken Enchiladas

Yield: 8 servings (serving size: 1 enchilada and ½ cup lettuce)

8   (6-inch) corn tortillas
Cooking spray
1½ tablespoons chopped onion
1½ tablespoons chopped fresh cilantro
1   jalapeño pepper, seeded and chopped
3   cups shredded cooked chicken breast
3   (10-ounce) cans enchilada sauce, divided
1½ cups (6 ounces) shredded reduced-fat sharp Cheddar cheese
½   cup diced tomato
⅓   cup sliced ripe olives
4   cups shredded iceberg lettuce

Wrap tortillas in aluminum foil; bake at 350° for 15 minutes. While tortillas bake, coat a large nonstick skillet with cooking spray; place over medium-high heat until hot. Add onion, cilantro, and pepper; sauté until onion is tender. Add chicken and 1 can enchilada sauce; cook 5 minutes.

Spoon chicken mixture evenly down centers of tortillas. Roll up tortillas; place, seam sides down, in a 13- x 9-inch baking dish. Heat remaining 2 cans enchilada sauce in a saucepan; pour over enchiladas, and top with cheese. Bake at 350° for 10 minutes or until enchiladas are thoroughly heated and cheese melts. Sprinkle evenly with tomato and olives. Serve over lettuce.

Per Serving:

Calories 272

Fat 9.7g (sat 3.1g)

Protein 24.7g

Carbohydrate 21.0g

Fiber 2.0g

Cholesterol 59mg

Sodium 597mg

Exchanges: 1 Starch, 1 Vegetable, 3 Lean Meat

Sweet-and-Sour Chicken

Yield: 6 servings

2   tablespoons cornstarch
2   tablespoons granulated brown sugar substitute
       (such as brown Sugar Twin)
¾   teaspoon ground ginger
¼   teaspoon garlic powder
1½ cups pineapple juice
¼   cup rice wine vinegar
¼   cup low-sodium soy sauce
¼   cup reduced-calorie ketchup
1   tablespoon low-sodium Worcestershire sauce
Cooking spray
1¼ pounds skinned, boned chicken breast halves,
       cut into 1-inch pieces
1   cup thinly sliced green pepper
3   cups cooked long-grain rice (cooked without salt or fat)

Combine first 9 ingredients; set aside.

Coat a large nonstick skillet with cooking spray; place over medium-high heat until hot. Add chicken; stir-fry 5 minutes. Add green pepper; stir-fry 2 minutes. Gradually stir cornstarch mixture into chicken mixture. Cook over medium heat, stirring constantly, until mixture is thickened and bubbly.

To serve, spoon ½ cup rice onto each plate; top evenly with chicken mixture.

Per Serving:

Calories 265	Fiber 0.8g
Fat 1.7g (sat 0.3g)	Cholesterol 55mg
Protein 24.4g	Sodium 402mg
Carbohydrate 35.9g	Exchanges: 2 Starch, 1 Vegetable, 2 Very Lean Meat

Chicken and Snow Pea Stir-Fry

Yield: 4 servings

Cooking spray
2   teaspoons vegetable oil, divided
¾   cup thinly sliced sweet red pepper (about 1 medium)
¾   cup thinly sliced sweet yellow pepper (about 1 medium)
6   ounces fresh snow pea pods
4   (4-ounce) skinned, boned chicken breast halves, cut into thin strips
1   clove garlic, minced
1   cup low-sodium chicken broth
¼   cup low-sodium soy sauce
1   tablespoon plus 1 teaspoon cornstarch
3   tablespoons dry sherry
1   teaspoon peeled, grated gingerroot
¼   cup sesame seeds, toasted
3   cups cooked long-grain rice (cooked without salt or fat)

Coat a large nonstick skillet with cooking spray. Add 1 teaspoon oil; place over medium-high heat until hot. Add peppers; stir-fry 2 minutes. Add snow peas; stir-fry 2 minutes. Remove from skillet; keep warm.

Add remaining oil to skillet. Add chicken and garlic; stir-fry 4 minutes or until chicken is lightly browned. Remove from skillet.

Combine broth and next 4 ingredients; stir well. Add chicken, broth mixture, and sesame seeds to skillet; stir-fry 3 minutes or until mixture is thickened and bubbly. Stir in vegetable mixture. To serve, spoon ¾ cup rice onto each plate; top evenly with chicken mixture.

Per Serving:

Calories 388	Fiber 3.0g
Fat 8.3g (sat 1.3g)	Cholesterol 49mg
Protein 26.7g	Sodium 472mg
Carbohydrate 46.3g	Exchanges: 3 Starch, 3 Lean Meat

Apple-Sesame Chicken

Yield: 2 servings

1   tablespoon reduced-calorie margarine
2   (4-ounce) skinned, boned chicken breast halves,
        cut into thin strips
3   cups fresh broccoli flowerets
1   cup cubed Red Delicious apple (about 1 medium)
¾   cup sliced fresh mushrooms
¼   cup thinly sliced celery
1   tablespoon water
¼   teaspoon salt
¼   teaspoon curry powder
1½   cups cooked long-grain rice (cooked without salt or fat)
½   teaspoon sesame seeds, toasted

Melt margarine in a large nonstick skillet over medium-high heat. Add chicken; stir-fry 3 minutes. Add broccoli and next 6 ingredients; cover, reduce heat, and simmer 5 minutes or until vegetables are crisp-tender, stirring often.

To serve, spoon ¾ cup rice onto each plate; top evenly with chicken mixture. Sprinkle with sesame seeds.

Per Serving:

Calories 391	Fiber 4.2g
Fat 6.2g (sat 1.0g)	Cholesterol 66mg
Protein 33.2g	Sodium 453mg
Carbohydrate 51.3g	Exchanges: 2 Starch, 1 Vegetable, 1 Fruit, 3 Very Lean Meat

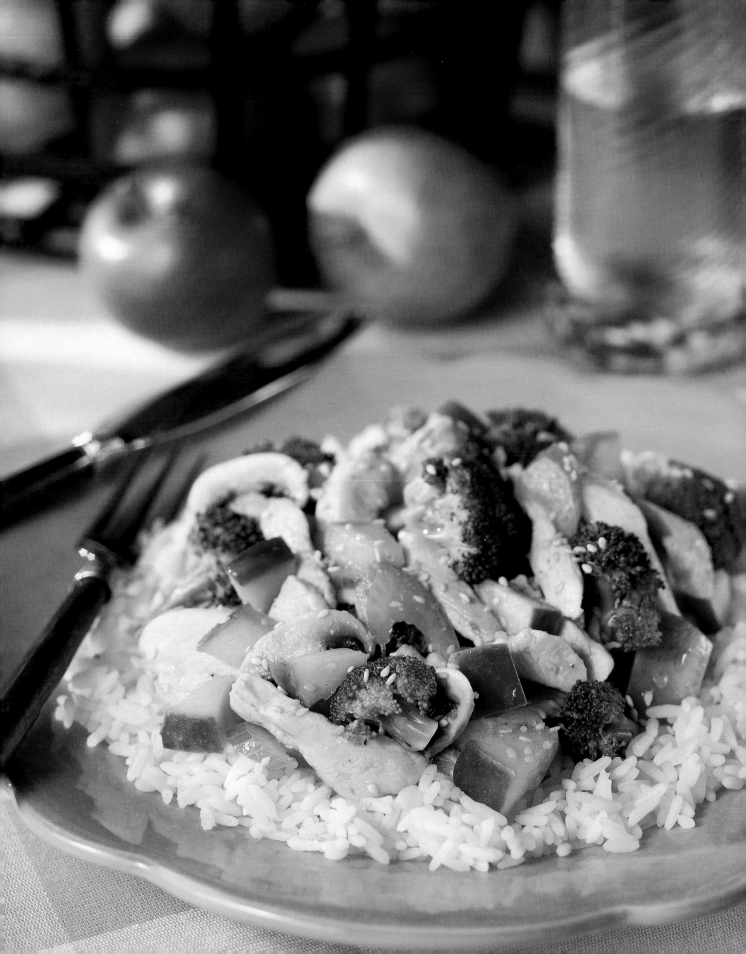

Chicken-Sausage Jambalaya

Yield: 6 (1½-cup) servings

¾ pound skinned, boned chicken breast halves, cut into pieces
½ teaspoon pepper
Olive oil-flavored cooking spray
1 teaspoon olive oil
10 ounces turkey breakfast sausage
2½ cups chopped onion (about 2 large)
2¼ cups chopped celery (about 6 stalks)
1¾ cups sliced green onions (about 7)
1 cup chopped green pepper
2 cloves garlic, minced
2 chicken-flavored bouillon cubes
3⅓ cups hot water
3 tablespoons fat-free Italian salad dressing
1¼ cups long-grain rice, uncooked

Sprinkle chicken with pepper. Coat a Dutch oven with cooking spray; add oil. Place over medium-high heat until hot. Add chicken; sauté 3 minutes. Remove chicken; set aside.

Combine sausage and next 5 ingredients in Dutch oven. Cook over medium-high heat until sausage is browned. Stir in chicken.

Dissolve bouillon cubes in hot water; stir in dressing. Add to Dutch oven, and bring to a boil. Stir in rice. Cover, reduce heat, and simmer 20 minutes or until rice is tender and liquid is absorbed. Toss before serving.

Per Serving:

Calories 345	Fiber 3.6g
Fat 7.5g (sat 1.2g)	Cholesterol 62mg
Protein 26.0g	Sodium 722mg
Carbohydrate 43.8g	Exchanges: 3 Starch, 3 Lean Meat

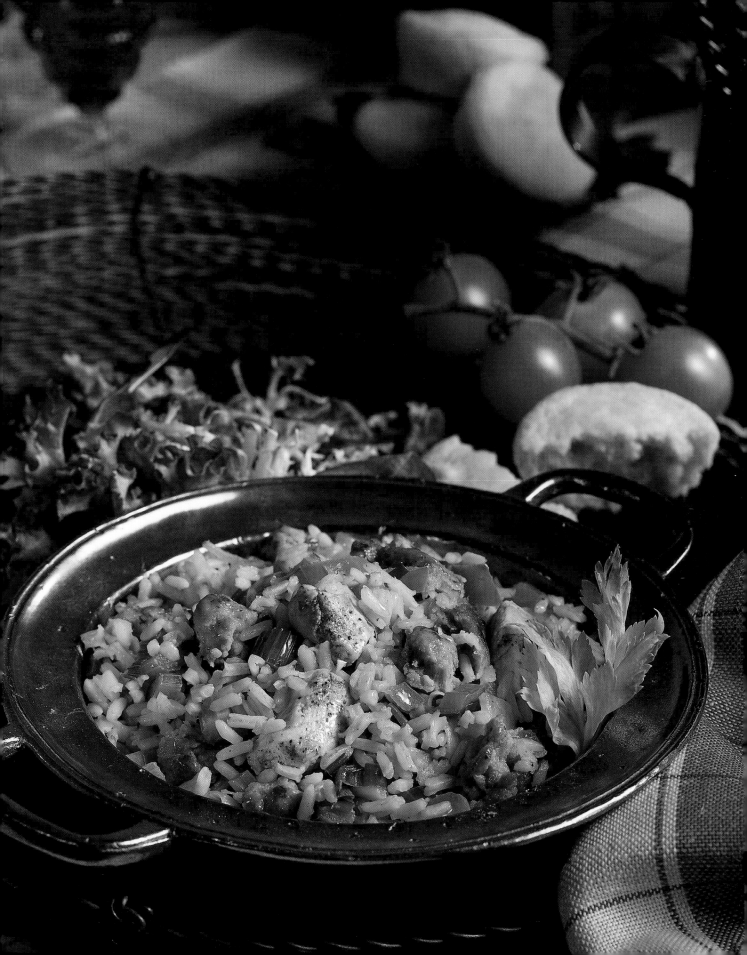

Chicken in Mustard Sauce

Yield: 4 servings

½   teaspoon paprika
¼   teaspoon salt
¼   teaspoon coarsely ground pepper
4   (4-ounce) skinned, boned chicken breast halves
Cooking spray
¼   cup dry white wine or low-sodium chicken broth
1½   tablespoons all-purpose flour
¾   cup 1% low-fat milk, divided
1   tablespoon peppercorn mustard (or regular prepared mustard)

Combine first 3 ingredients; sprinkle over chicken. Coat a nonstick skillet with cooking spray; place over medium-high heat until hot. Add chicken; cook 3 to 5 minutes on each side, or until browned. Remove chicken from skillet, and set aside.

Add wine (or broth) to skillet; deglaze by scraping particles that cling to bottom. Combine flour and ¼ cup milk, stirring until smooth; add to skillet. Stir in remaining ½ cup milk and mustard. Cook over medium heat, stirring constantly, until thickened. Return chicken to skillet. Bring to a boil; cover, reduce heat, and simmer 5 minutes or until chicken is done. Serve chicken with sauce.

Per Serving:

Calories 163	**Fiber** 0.2g
Fat 2.4g (sat 0.7g)	**Cholesterol** 68mg
Protein 28.1g	**Sodium** 356mg
Carbohydrate 5.1g	**Exchanges:** 4 Very Lean Meat

If you like a powerful mustard punch, add an extra tablespoon of mustard.

Citrus-Ginger Chicken

Yield: 4 servings

2½ tablespoons low-sugar orange marmalade
⅛ teaspoon grated lime rind
1½ tablespoons fresh lime juice
1½ teaspoons peeled, grated gingerroot
Cooking spray
4 (6-ounce) skinned chicken breast halves

Combine first 4 ingredients in a small bowl.

Coat grill rack with cooking spray; place on grill over medium-hot coals (350° to 400°). Place chicken on rack; grill, covered, 20 to 25 minutes or until done, turning and basting with marmalade mixture.

Per Serving:

Calories 147	Fiber 0.0g
Fat 3.2g (sat 0.9g)	Cholesterol 72mg
Protein 26.5g	Sodium 64mg
Carbohydrate 1.3g	Exchanges: 4 Very Lean Meat

(Photograph on page 117)

Fresh lime and ginger give this easy grilled chicken real zing.

Baked Buffalo Chicken

Yield: 4 servings (serving size: 2 thighs plus 2 tablespoons dressing)

Cooking spray
1½ teaspoons vegetable oil
8 small chicken thighs (about 1½ pounds), skinned
¼ cup hot sauce
3 tablespoons fat-free margarine, melted
2 tablespoons water
1 tablespoon white vinegar
1 teaspoon celery seeds
⅛ teaspoon pepper
½ cup fat-free blue cheese salad dressing

Coat a nonstick skillet with cooking spray; add oil. Place over medium-high heat until hot. Add chicken; cook 4 minutes on each side. Transfer chicken to an 11- x 7-inch baking dish coated with cooking spray.

Combine hot sauce and next 5 ingredients; pour over chicken. Bake, uncovered, at 400° for 25 minutes. Serve with blue cheese dressing.

Per Serving:

Calories 212	Fiber 0.7g
Fat 6.7g (sat 1.5g)	Cholesterol 95mg
Protein 23.2g	Sodium 575mg
Carbohydrate 11.6g	Exchanges: 1 Starch, 3 Lean Meat

These chicken thighs may remind you of the spicy chicken wings served at your local sports grill. You'll need the cool blue cheese dressing to tame the heat.

Lemon-Roasted Chicken

Yield: 4 servings

1½ teaspoons salt
2 teaspoons freshly ground pepper
2 to 3 teaspoons dried rosemary, crushed
1 (3-pound) broiler-fryer
1 medium lemon, cut in half
Cooking spray

Combine first 3 ingredients; set aside.

Loosen skin from chicken breast by running fingers between the two; rub 1 teaspoon seasoning mixture under skin. Rub remaining mixture over outside of chicken. Place chicken in a heavy-duty, zip-top plastic bag; seal and refrigerate 8 hours.

Remove chicken from bag. Insert lemon halves in cavity; tie ends of legs together with string. Lift wing tips up and over back, and tuck under bird. Place chicken, breast side down, in a roasting pan coated with cooking spray.

Bake, uncovered, at 450° for 50 minutes or until a meat thermometer inserted in thigh registers 180°. Let stand 10 minutes before serving.

Per Serving:

Calories 225	Fiber 0.5g
Fat 8.6g (sat 2.3g)	Cholesterol 101mg
Protein 33.3g	Sodium 978mg
Carbohydrate 3.9g	Exchanges: 4 Lean Meat

Roast the chicken with the skin on to keep it moist, but be sure to remove the skin before you eat it because it contains a lot of fat.

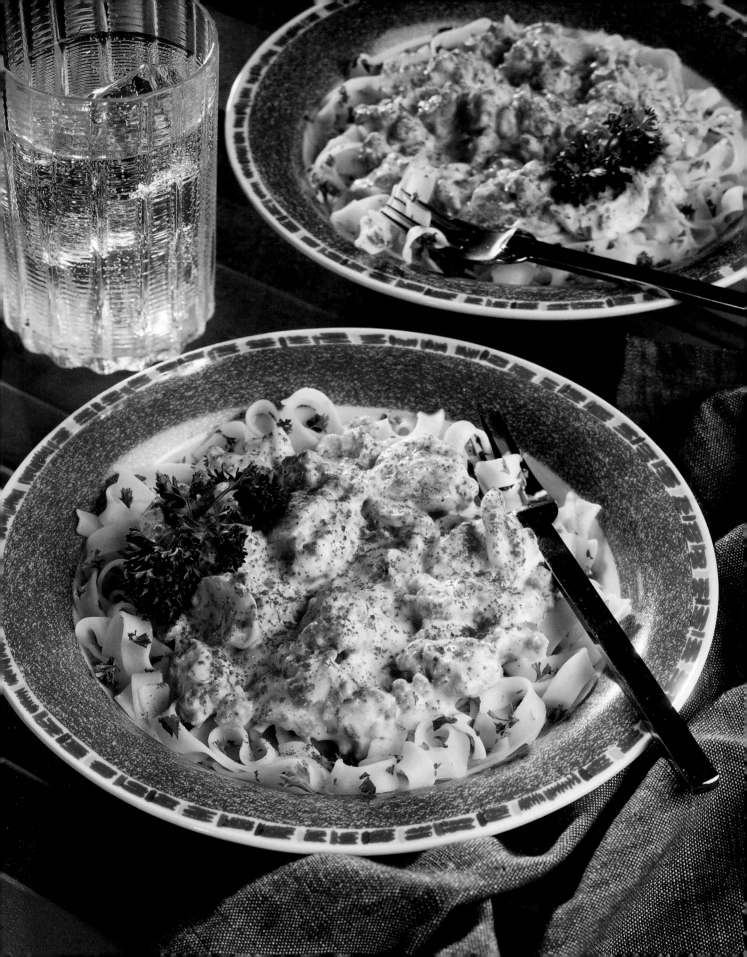

Turkey Stroganoff

Yield: 4 servings

8   ounces medium egg noodles, uncooked
1   tablespoon chopped fresh parsley
Cooking spray
1   pound freshly ground raw turkey
½   cup chopped onion
1½ cups sliced fresh mushrooms
⅓   cup dry white wine or low-sodium chicken broth
¼   teaspoon salt
⅛   teaspoon ground nutmeg
⅛   teaspoon freshly ground pepper
1   cup 1% low-fat cottage cheese
½   cup fat-free sour cream
1   tablespoon lemon juice
Hungarian paprika

Cook noodles according to package directions, omitting salt and fat. Drain; toss with parsley.

Coat a nonstick skillet with cooking spray; place over medium heat until hot. Add turkey and onion; cook until turkey is browned. Add mushrooms and next 4 ingredients. Cook over low heat 10 minutes or until liquid evaporates, stirring occasionally. Remove from heat.

Combine cottage cheese, sour cream, and lemon juice in container of an electric blender; cover and process until smooth. Add to turkey mixture; cook over low heat, stirring constantly, until thoroughly heated. Serve over noodles. Sprinkle with paprika.

Per Serving:

Calories 440	Fiber 2.0g
Fat 6.5g (sat 2.0g)	Cholesterol 130mg
Protein 42.4g	Sodium 491mg
Carbohydrate 47.0g	Exchanges: 3 Starch, 5 Very Lean Meat

Turkey Parmesan

Yield: 4 servings

1   egg, lightly beaten
2   teaspoons vegetable oil
½   cup Italian-seasoned breadcrumbs
2   tablespoons grated Parmesan cheese
1   pound turkey breast cutlets
Cooking spray
½   cup low-fat marinara sauce or pasta sauce

Combine egg and oil in a shallow dish. Combine breadcrumbs and cheese in a shallow dish. Dip cutlets in egg mixture; dredge in breadcrumb mixture. Place cutlets on a baking sheet coated with cooking spray.

Coat cutlets lightly with cooking spray. Bake at 350° for 12 to 15 minutes or until done.

Place marinara sauce in a microwave-safe bowl. Cover and microwave at MEDIUM-HIGH (70% power) 2 minutes or until thoroughly heated, stirring once. Spoon warm sauce over cutlets. Serve immediately.

Per Serving:

Calories 273	Fiber 0.6g
Fat 8.1g (sat 2.2g)	Cholesterol 123mg
Protein 32.7g	Sodium 678mg
Carbohydrate 15.2g	Exchanges: 1 Starch, 4 Lean Meat

You'll have an Italian-inspired classic on the table in less than 30 minutes with this super-quick entrée.

Salads

Cabbage-Pineapple Slaw, page 145

Holiday Cranberry Salad

Yield: 5 (½-cup) servings

2 cups fresh or frozen cranberries, thawed
¼ cup granulated sugar substitute with aspartame (such as Equal Spoonful)
1 (0.3-ounce) package sugar-free lemon gelatin
1¼ cups boiling water
½ cup finely chopped celery (about 2 stalks)
1 cup finely chopped Granny Smith apple (about 1 medium)
Cooking spray
Green leaf lettuce (optional)

Position knife blade in food processor bowl; add cranberries. Process 30 seconds or until chopped. Combine cranberries and sugar substitute in a large bowl; let stand 30 minutes or until sugar substitute dissolves. Combine gelatin and boiling water in a large bowl; stir 2 minutes or until gelatin dissolves. Chill until the consistency of unbeaten egg white.

Stir cranberry mixture, celery, and apple into gelatin mixture. Pour mixture into a 3-cup mold coated with cooking spray. Cover and chill until firm.

To serve, unmold salad onto a lettuce-lined serving plate, if desired.

Per Serving:

Calories 50	Fiber 1.2g
Fat 0.8g (sat 0.0g)	Cholesterol 0mg
Protein 1.4g	Sodium 17mg
Carbohydrate 9.8g	Exchange: ½ Fruit

Antipasto Platter

Yield: 4 servings

1   (10-ounce) package frozen artichoke hearts
1½ cups small fresh mushrooms, halved
⅔   cup chopped purple onion
1   (15-ounce) can garbanzo beans (chick-peas), rinsed and drained
1   (15-ounce) can no-salt-added kidney beans, rinsed and drained
¾   cup reduced-fat olive oil vinaigrette, divided
6   cups torn romaine lettuce
4   ounces thinly sliced fat-free turkey ham, cut into thin strips
4   ounces part-skim mozzarella cheese, thinly sliced
2   medium-size sweet red peppers, seeded and thinly sliced
2   medium cucumbers, sliced

Cook artichoke hearts according to package directions, omitting salt and fat. Drain well.

Combine artichoke hearts, mushrooms, and next 3 ingredients in a large bowl; add ½ cup vinaigrette, and toss well. Cover and chill 2 hours, stirring occasionally.

Place romaine lettuce on a large serving platter; spoon artichoke mixture onto lettuce in center of platter. Arrange ham strips, cheese, sweet red pepper, and cucumber around artichoke mixture. Drizzle remaining vinaigrette over salad.

Per Serving:

Calories 316   Fiber 6.1g
Fat 12.0g (sat 3.0g)   Cholesterol 22mg
Protein 19.6g   Sodium 596mg
Carbohydrate 37.0g   Exchanges: 2 Starch, 1 Vegetable, 2 Medium-Fat Meat

In 1749, a Swedish explorer made note of an "unusual salad . . . that tastes better than one can imagine—cabbage—cut into long, thin strips." It was called koolsla, from the Dutch words for cabbage (kool) and salad (sla), thus coleslaw.

<u>Saveur</u>, January/February 1997

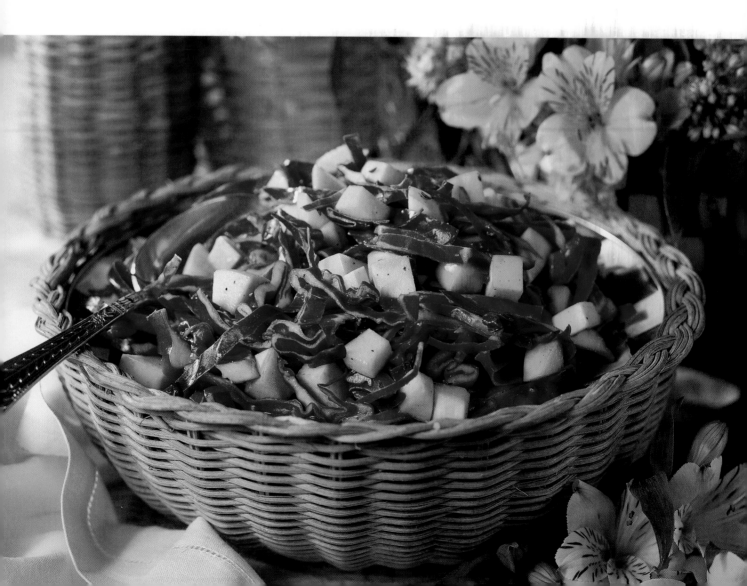

Apple Slaw

Yield: 6 (1-cup) servings

⅓	cup cider vinegar
2	teaspoons olive oil
1	teaspoon granulated sugar substitute (such as Sugar Twin)
1	teaspoon Dijon mustard
½	teaspoon caraway seeds
¼	teaspoon salt
¼	teaspoon pepper
7	cups shredded red cabbage
1½	cups diced Golden Delicious apple (about 2 medium)

Combine first 7 ingredients in a large bowl, stirring with a whisk until blended. Add cabbage and apple; toss well.

Cover and chill thoroughly, tossing occasionally.

Per Serving:

Calories 55	Fiber 2.1g
Fat 1.9g (sat 0.2g)	Cholesterol 0mg
Protein 1.1g	Sodium 132mg
Carbohydrate 10.0g	Exchanges: 1 Vegetable, ½ Fruit

Vinaigrette Coleslaw

Yield: 5 (½-cup) servings

3	cups finely shredded cabbage
¼	cup chopped sweet red pepper
2	tablespoons thinly sliced green onions
2	tablespoons chopped fresh parsley
¼	cup plus 2 tablespoons water
¼	cup white wine vinegar
1	tablespoon granulated sugar substitute (such as Sugar Twin)
2	teaspoons olive oil
¼	teaspoon freshly ground pepper
¼	teaspoon dried basil
⅛	teaspoon garlic powder

Combine first 4 ingredients in small bowl; toss well. Combine water and remaining 6 ingredients in a jar; cover tightly, and shake vigorously. Pour vinegar mixture over cabbage mixture. Cover and chill thoroughly.

Toss gently before serving. Serve with a slotted spoon.

Per Serving:

Calories 34	**Fiber** 1.3g
Fat 1.9g (sat 0.3g)	**Cholesterol** 0mg
Protein 0.7g	**Sodium** 13mg
Carbohydrate 3.6g	**Exchange:** 1 Vegetable

Cabbage-Pineapple Slaw

Yield: 5 (1-cup) servings

1   (8-ounce) can pineapple tidbits in juice, undrained
3   cups finely shredded cabbage
1½   cups chopped Red Delicious apple (about 2 medium)
½   cup chopped celery
¼   cup golden raisins
¼   cup reduced-fat mayonnaise
Cabbage leaves (optional)
Apple slices (optional)

Drain pineapple, reserving 3 tablespoons juice. Combine drained pineapple, shredded cabbage, and next 3 ingredients in a large bowl.

Combine reserved pineapple juice and mayonnaise; add to cabbage mixture, tossing gently. Cover and chill.

To serve, spoon mixture into a cabbage leaf-lined bowl, and garnish with apple slices, if desired.

Per Serving:

Calories 108	Fiber 2.9g
Fat 3.5g (sat 0.3g)	Cholesterol 4mg
Protein 1.2g	Sodium 109mg
Carbohydrate 20.2g	Exchanges: 1 Vegetable, 1 Fruit, 1 Fat

(Photograph on page 139)

This tasty chilled salad is a cross between Waldorf salad and coleslaw.

Tossed Salad with Buttermilk Dressing

Yield: 6 (½-cup) servings

2	cups tightly packed torn romaine lettuce
2	cups tightly packed torn leaf lettuce
1¼	cups halved cherry tomatoes
½	cup sliced purple onion
¼	cup chopped celery
½	cup nonfat buttermilk
¼	cup plus 2 tablespoons nonfat mayonnaise
1	tablespoon grated Parmesan cheese
1	teaspoon dried parsley flakes
¼	teaspoon cracked pepper
1	clove garlic, minced

Combine first 5 ingredients in a large bowl; toss well.

Combine buttermilk and remaining 5 ingredients in a small bowl; stir well. Spoon buttermilk dressing over salad; toss gently to coat. Serve immediately.

Per Serving:

Calories 42	Fiber 1.3g
Fat 0.5g (sat 0.3g)	Cholesterol 1mg
Protein 2.1g	Sodium 239mg
Carbohydrate 7.8g	Exchange: 1 Vegetable

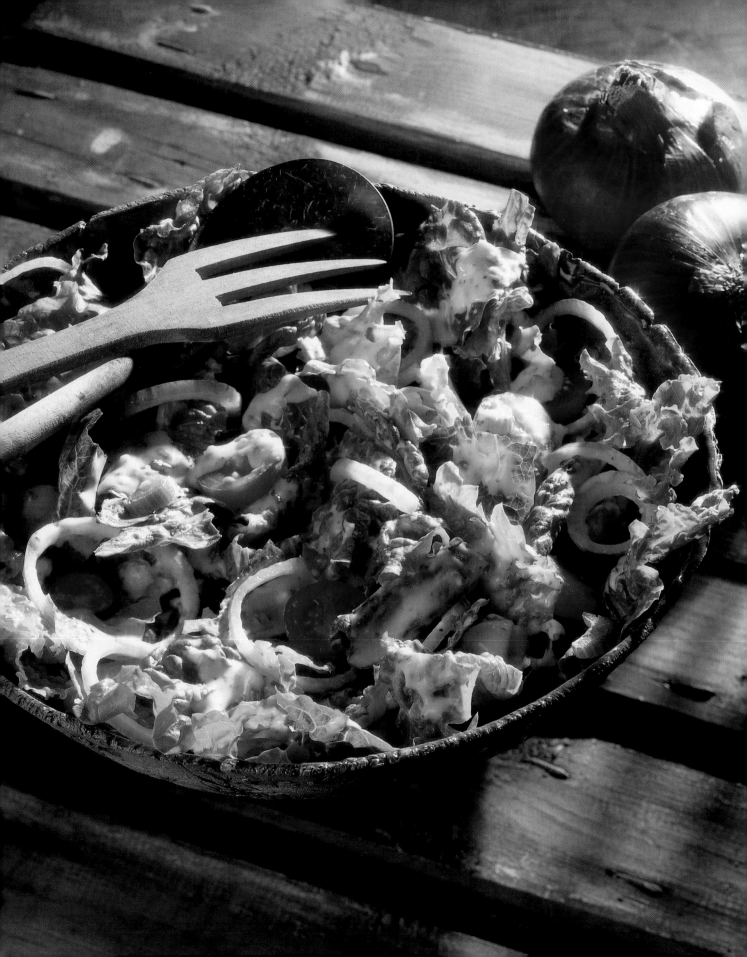

Spinach Salad with the Blues

Yield: 6 servings

⅓   cup fat-free, reduced-sodium chicken broth
¼   cup white wine vinegar
1   tablespoon prepared mustard
1   teaspoon granulated sugar substitute (such as Sugar Twin)
1   (10-ounce) package fresh spinach, washed, trimmed, and shredded
5   heads Belgian endive (about 10 ounces), washed and trimmed
2   Red Delicious apples, cored and thinly sliced
¼   cup chopped walnuts, toasted
1   (4-ounce) package crumbled blue cheese

Combine first 4 ingredients in a jar. Cover tightly, and shake vigorously.

Combine spinach and dressing in a large bowl, tossing gently. Divide spinach mixture evenly among six salad plates. Arrange endive leaves and apple slices beside spinach mixture.

To serve, sprinkle evenly with walnuts and blue cheese.

Per Serving:

Calories 159	**Fiber** 4.1g
Fat 8.7g (sat 3.8g)	**Cholesterol** 14mg
Protein 7.0g	**Sodium** 331mg
Carbohydrate 15.4g	**Exchanges:** 1 Vegetable, ½ Fruit, 1 High-Fat Meat

If you're a true blue cheese lover, this salad will become one of your favorites.

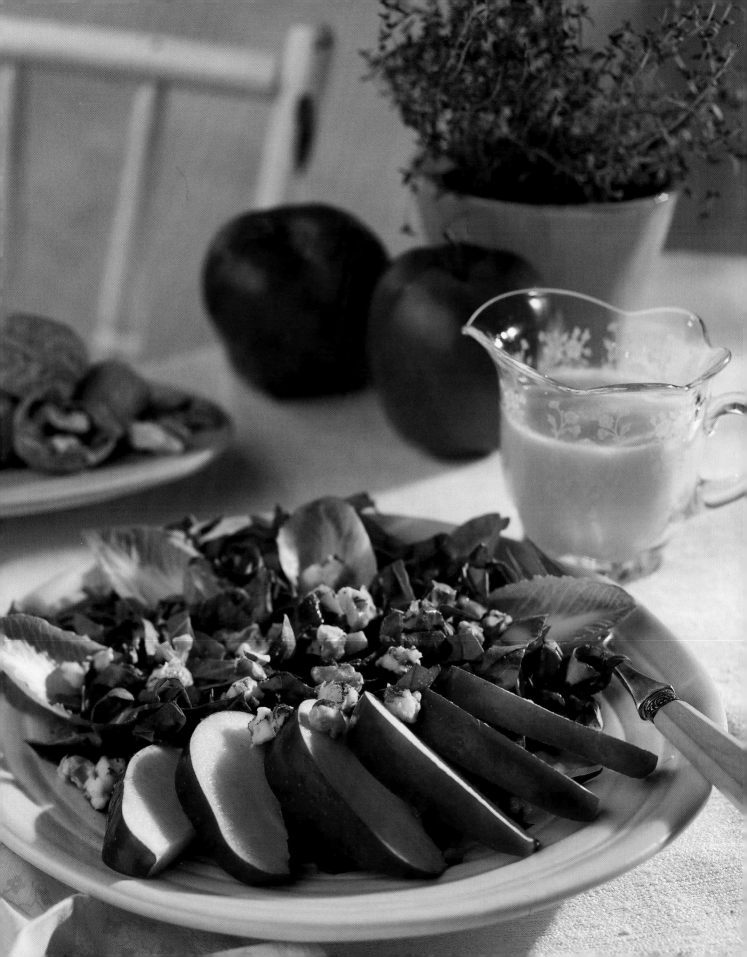

Broccoli Salad

Yield: 9 (¾-cup) servings

½	cup raisins
1	(1-pound) bag broccoli flowerets, chopped
1	cup seedless grapes, halved
3	green onions, thinly sliced
⅔	cup reduced-fat mayonnaise
2	tablespoons tarragon vinegar
2	tablespoons slivered almonds, toasted
4	slices turkey bacon, cooked and crumbled

Soak raisins in hot water to cover 5 minutes; drain.

Combine raisins and next 3 ingredients in a large bowl. Combine mayonnaise and vinegar; stir into broccoli mixture. Cover and chill.

Stir in almonds and bacon just before serving.

Per Serving:

Calories 129	Fiber 2.1g
Fat 7.5g (sat 1.1g)	Cholesterol 10mg
Protein 3.1g	Sodium 222mg
Carbohydrate 14.7g	Exchanges: ½ Fruit, 1 Vegetable, 1½ Fat

Sweet and savory, creamy and crunchy—this all-purpose salad is one of our favorites.

Corn Salad

Yield: 8 (½-cup) servings

2 (11-ounce) cans white shoepeg corn, drained
1 green pepper, chopped
½ cup chopped purple onion
½ cup fat-free sour cream
1 tablespoon white vinegar
¼ teaspoon celery salt
⅛ teaspoon pepper

Combine all ingredients in a medium bowl, stirring well. Cover and chill at least 3 hours.

Serve with a slotted spoon.

Per Serving:

Calories 71

Fat 0.4g (sat 0.1g)

Protein 2.9g

Carbohydrate 15.8g

Fiber 1.0g

Cholesterol 0mg

Sodium 257mg

Exchange: 1 Starch

This colorful salad is great for pot-luck dinners and covered-dish functions.

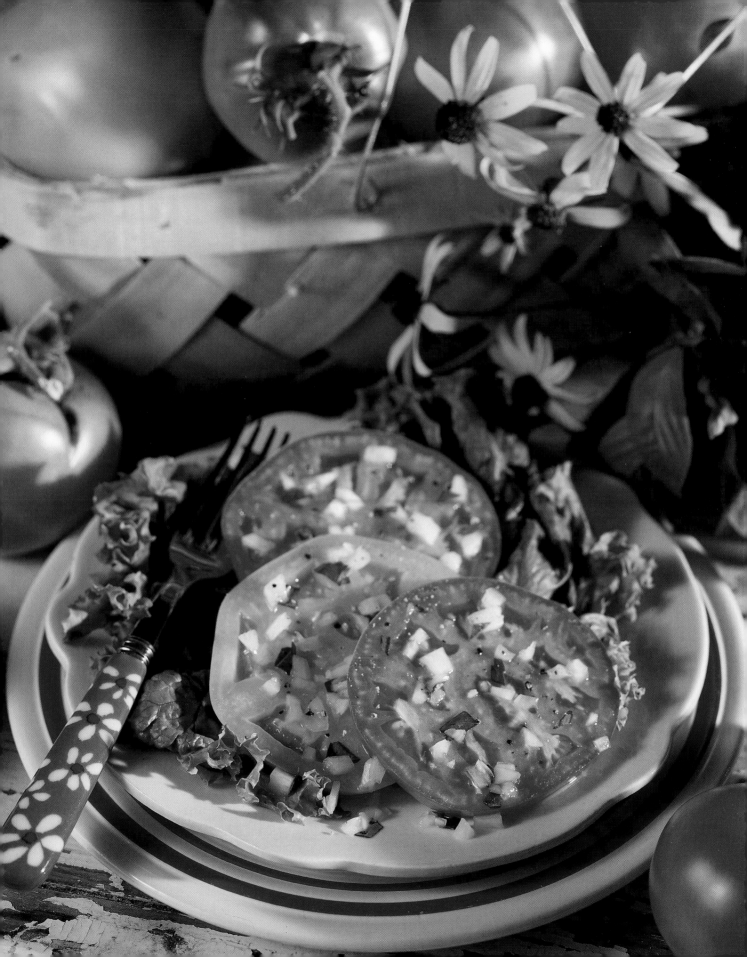

Marinated Tomato Slices

Yield: 8 servings

4   large red or yellow tomatoes, cut into ¼-inch slices
¼   cup lemon juice
2   tablespoons minced purple onion
2   tablespoons red wine vinegar
1   tablespoon chopped fresh basil or 1 teaspoon dried basil
¼   teaspoon freshly ground pepper
1   clove garlic, minced
Green leaf lettuce leaves (optional)

Arrange tomato slices in a large shallow dish. Combine lemon juice and next 5 ingredients; pour over tomato slices, turning to coat. Cover and marinate in refrigerator at least 2 hours.

Arrange tomato slices evenly on 8 lettuce-lined salad plates, if desired. Spoon marinade evenly over tomato slices.

Per Serving:

Calories 25	Fiber 1.4g
Fat 0.3g (sat 0.0g)	Cholesterol 0mg
Protein 1.0g	Sodium 9mg
Carbohydrate 5.9g	Exchange: 1 Vegetable

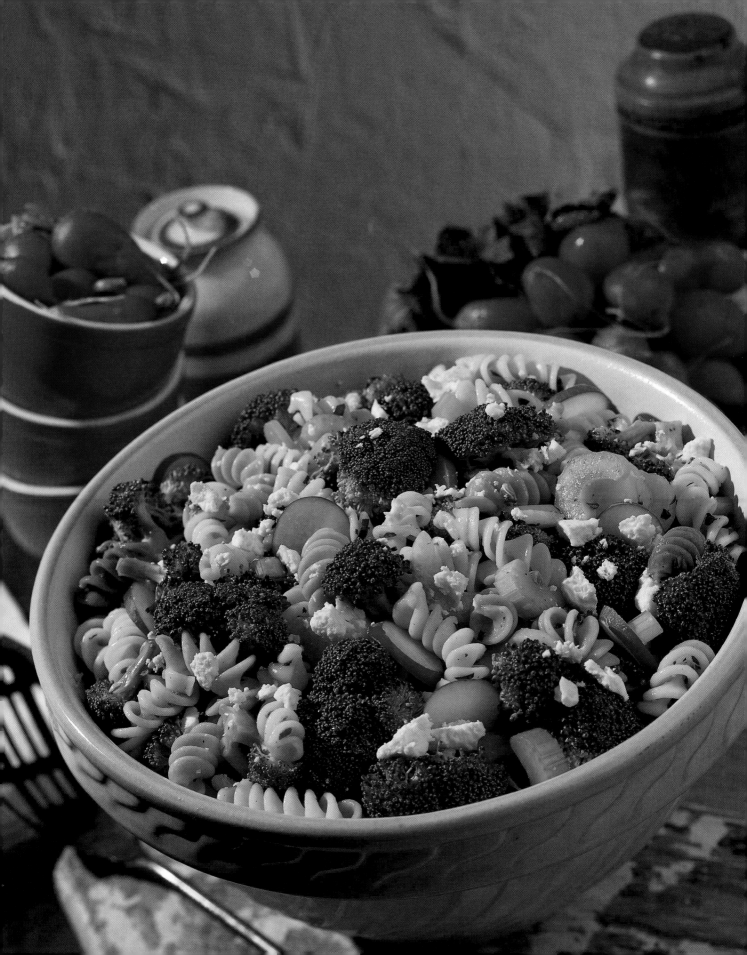

Pasta-Vegetable Salad

Yield: 11 (1-cup) servings

6	ounces tricolor rotini pasta, uncooked
1	(1-pound) bag broccoli flowerets
3	stalks celery, sliced
1	(8-ounce) can sliced water chestnuts, drained
1	(1.05-ounce) package fat-free Italian dressing mix
3	tablespoons chopped fresh oregano
¾	cup sliced radishes
⅓	cup crumbled reduced-fat feta cheese

Prepare pasta according to package directions, omitting salt and fat; drain. Rinse with cold water; drain.

Combine pasta, broccoli, celery, and water chestnuts in a bowl; set aside.

Prepare dressing mix according to package directions; stir in oregano. Pour over pasta mixture, stirring to coat. Cover and chill at least 6 hours, stirring occasionally. Just before serving, stir in radishes, and sprinkle with cheese.

Per Serving:

Calories 101	Fiber 0.7g
Fat 1.0g (sat 0.3g)	Cholesterol 2mg
Protein 3.5g	Sodium 281mg
Carbohydrate 19.6g	Exchanges: 1 Starch, 1 Vegetable

Add the radishes to the salad just before serving. Otherwise, their red color will bleed onto the pasta and vegetables.

Ham and Potato Salad

Yield: 6 (1½-cup) servings

1	pound small round red potatoes, cut into ½-inch slices (about 3 cups)
1	(16-ounce) package frozen mixed vegetables
⅓	cup reduced-fat mayonnaise
⅓	cup fat-free sour cream
½	cup sliced green onions
½	teaspoon pepper
1½	cups diced lean cooked ham

Place potato in boiling water to cover; cover, reduce heat, and cook 10 minutes or until tender (do not overcook). Drain and set aside.

Cook frozen mixed vegetables according to package directions, omitting salt and fat; drain and set aside.

Combine mayonnaise and next 3 ingredients in a large bowl. Gently stir in potato, vegetables, and ham. Cover and chill at least 8 hours.

Per Serving:

Calories 207	Fiber 4.4g
Fat 6.1g (sat 1.3g)	Cholesterol 30mg
Protein 13.1g	Sodium 729mg
Carbohydrate 25.2g	Exchanges: 1 Starch, 1 Vegetable, 1 Lean Meat, ½ Fat

Shrimp Salad

Yield: 2 (1-cup) servings

1	pound unpeeled medium-size fresh shrimp
3	cups water
⅓	cup fat-free sour cream
2	tablespoons finely chopped celery
1	tablespoon finely chopped onion
2	teaspoons lemon juice
⅛	teaspoon salt
⅛	teaspoon curry powder
2	green lettuce leaves

Peel and devein shrimp. Bring water to a boil; add shrimp, and cook 3 to 5 minutes or until shrimp turn pink. Drain well; rinse with cold water. Cut each shrimp in half crosswise, and place in a small bowl.

Combine sour cream and next 5 ingredients, stirring well. Add sour cream mixture to shrimp, and toss gently. Cover and chill thoroughly.

Serve on lettuce-lined plates.

Per Serving:

Calories 148	Fiber 0.6g
Fat 1.3g (sat 0.3g)	Cholesterol 221mg
Protein 26.8g	Sodium 438mg
Carbohydrate 4.7g	Exchanges: 1 Vegetable, 3 Very Lean Meat

You can put everything, and the
more things the better, into a salad,
as into a conversation; but everything
depends on the skill of mixing.

CHARLES DUDLEY WARNER, American writer

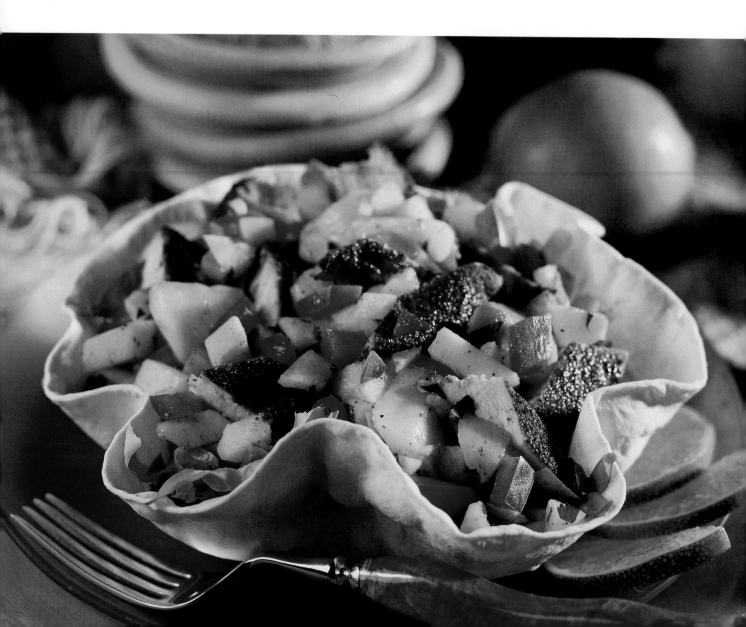

Chicken Taco Salad

Yield: 4 servings

4   (4-ounce) skinned, boned chicken breast halves
2   tablespoons salt-free Mexican seasoning, divided
4   (10-inch) flour tortillas
Cooking spray
½   cup chopped green pepper
½   cup chopped sweet red pepper
½   cup chopped jicama
1   tablespoon chopped fresh cilantro
1   medium mango, peeled and chopped
2   tablespoons water
2   tablespoons lime juice
2   teaspoons vegetable oil
1   teaspoon granulated sugar substitute (such as Sugar Twin)
6   cups shredded Bibb lettuce
Lime slices (optional)

Coat chicken with 1 tablespoon Mexican seasoning. Cover and refrigerate 8 hours.

Press each tortilla into a small microwave-safe bowl; microwave at HIGH 1½ minutes or until crisp.

Coat a nonstick skillet with cooking spray; place over medium heat. Add chicken; cook 5 minutes on each side or until done. Chop chicken. Combine chicken, peppers, and next 3 ingredients. Combine remaining 1 tablespoon Mexican seasoning, water, and next 3 ingredients; drizzle over chicken mixture; toss well. Arrange lettuce evenly in tortilla bowls; top with chicken mixture. Serve with lime slices, if desired.

Per Serving:

Calories 378	Fiber 4.2g
Fat 8.2g (sat 1.5g)	Cholesterol 66mg
Protein 32.4g	Sodium 341mg
Carbohydrate 43.5g	Exchanges: 3 Starch, 3 Lean Meat

Chicken and Fettuccine Salad

Yield: 8 (1-cup) servings

6   ounces uncooked fettuccine, broken in half
2½   cups broccoli flowerets
1   cup diagonally sliced carrot
¾   cup diagonally sliced celery
⅓   cup fat-free Italian dressing
⅓   cup low-fat mayonnaise
2½   tablespoons prepared horseradish
½   teaspoon freshly ground pepper
2½   cups chopped cooked chicken breast
12   cherry tomatoes, halved

Cook fettuccine according to package directions, omitting salt and fat. Drain and rinse under cold water; drain again. Set aside.

Cook broccoli, carrot, and celery in a small amount of boiling water 6 minutes or until crisp-tender. Drain; plunge into ice water, and drain again.

Combine cooked fettuccine and broccoli mixture in a large bowl. Combine Italian dressing and next 3 ingredients; stir well. Add to fettuccine mixture; toss gently. Stir in chicken and tomato.

Per Serving:

Calories 196	Fiber 3.7g
Fat 4.7g (sat 0.9g)	Cholesterol 39mg
Protein 17.6g	Sodium 238mg
Carbohydrate 22.2g	Exchanges: 1 Starch, 1 Vegetable, 2 Lean Meat

French-Style Green Beans, page 166

Sides

Asparagus with Garlic Cream • Lemon-Dill Carrots

Oriental Broccoli • French-Style Green Beans • Corn Pudding

Okra-Tomato-Zucchini Medley • Crispy Onion Rings

Pretty Pepper Kabobs • Chili-Fried Potatoes

New Potatoes with Chives • Brown Rice Pilaf • Southwestern Rice

Vermicelli with Tomato Basil • Tangy Dijon Pasta

Sausage-Cornbread Dressing

Asparagus with Garlic Cream

Yield: 8 servings

1	(8-ounce) carton reduced-fat sour cream
3	tablespoons fat-free milk
1	tablespoon white wine vinegar
⅛	teaspoon salt
⅛	teaspoon freshly ground pepper
2	cloves garlic, minced
2	pounds fresh asparagus
2	teaspoons chopped fresh chives

Combine first 6 ingredients, stirring well. Cover and chill at least 2 hours.

Snap off tough ends of asparagus; remove scales from stalks with a vegetable peeler, if desired.

Place asparagus in a small amount of boiling water. Cover, reduce heat, and cook 4 minutes or until crisp-tender; drain. Plunge into ice water to stop the cooking process; drain. Cover and chill.

To serve, place asparagus on a serving platter. Top with sauce, and sprinkle with chives.

Per Serving:

Calories 58	Fiber 1.5g
Fat 3.6g (sat 2.2g)	Cholesterol 11mg
Protein 2.7g	Sodium 51mg
Carbohydrate 5.0g	Exchanges: 1 Vegetable, 1 Fat

Drizzle crisp-tender asparagus spears with a garlicky cream sauce and top with a sprinkling of fragrant snipped chives.

Lemon-Dill Carrots

Yield: 8 (½-cup) servings

8	medium carrots, scraped and diagonally sliced
1	teaspoon cornstarch
1	tablespoon lemon juice
⅓	cup water
1	teaspoon margarine
½	teaspoon dried dillweed
¼	teaspoon grated lemon rind
⅛	teaspoon salt

Arrange carrot in a vegetable steamer over boiling water. Cover; steam 2 to 3 minutes or until crisp-tender. Transfer carrot to a serving bowl, and keep warm.

Combine cornstarch and lemon juice in a small saucepan, stirring until smooth. Add water; cook over medium heat, stirring constantly, until thickened.

Stir in margarine and next 3 ingredients. Cook, stirring constantly, until margarine melts.

To serve, pour lemon juice mixture over carrot, and toss gently.

Per Serving:

Calories 41	Fiber 2.6g
Fat 0.6g (sat 0.1g)	Cholesterol 0mg
Protein 0.9g	Sodium 71mg
Carbohydrate 8.8g	Exchange: 1 Vegetable

Oriental Broccoli

Yield: 6 (1-cup) servings

1½ pounds fresh broccoli
3   tablespoons low-sodium soy sauce
2   teaspoons dark sesame oil
1   teaspoon honey
½   teaspoon peeled, grated gingerroot or ¼ teaspoon ground ginger
¼   teaspoon dry mustard
8   small cherry tomatoes, halved
½   cup sliced water chestnuts
2   green onions, diagonally sliced

Trim off large leaves of broccoli, and remove tough ends of lower stalks. Wash broccoli thoroughly, and coarsely chop. Arrange in a vegetable steamer over boiling water. Cover and steam 5 to 8 minutes or until crisp-tender. Drain; transfer to a serving bowl, and keep warm.

Combine soy sauce and next 4 ingredients in a small saucepan; stir well. Bring to a boil over medium heat. Pour over broccoli. Add tomato, water chestnuts, and green onions; toss gently. Serve immediately.

Per Serving:

Calories 56

Fat 1.9g (sat 0.3g)

Protein 3.1g

Carbohydrate 8.2g

Fiber 3.2g

Cholesterol 0mg

Sodium 223mg

Exchanges: 2 Vegetable

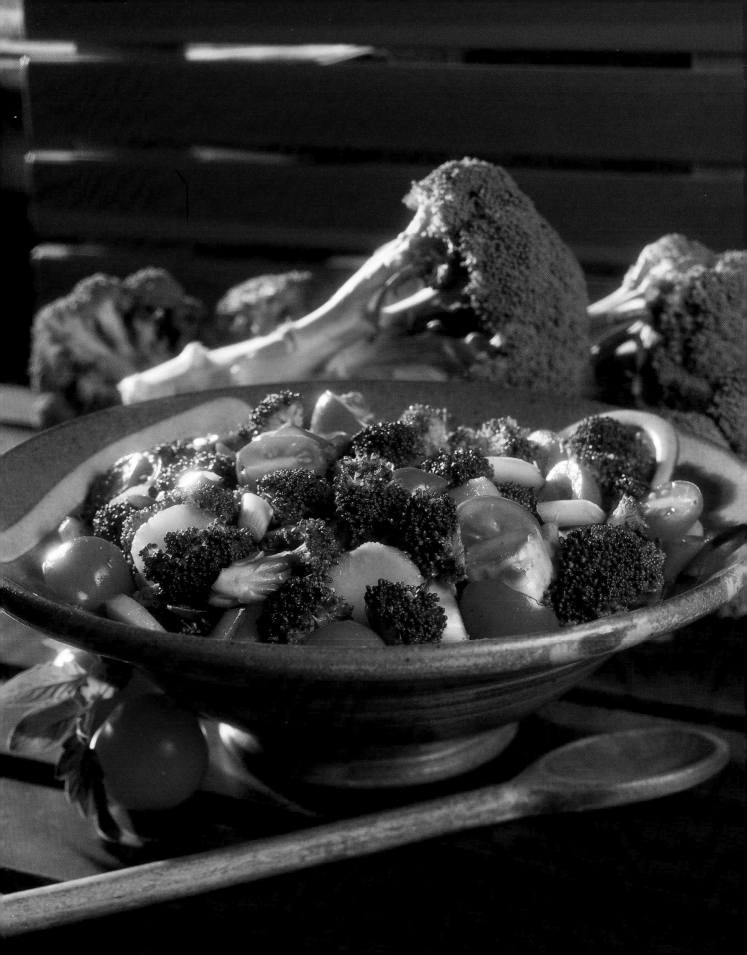

French-Style Green Beans

Yield: 4 (½-cup) servings

¾   pound fresh green beans, ends trimmed and strings removed
1   tablespoon fat-free margarine
¾   cup low-sodium chicken broth
¼   teaspoon freshly ground pepper
⅛   teaspoon salt
1½   teaspoons cornstarch
1   tablespoon water
2   teaspoons lemon juice
2   tablespoons sliced almonds, toasted

Slice beans in half lengthwise. Melt margarine in a large skillet. Add beans, and sauté 5 minutes. Add chicken broth, pepper, and salt. Bring to a boil. Cover, reduce heat, and simmer 15 minutes.

Combine cornstarch and water; pour over beans. Cook, tossing gently, 1 minute. Stir in lemon juice. Just before serving, sprinkle with toasted almonds.

Per Serving:

Calories 49   Fiber 2.0g
Fat 1.3g (sat 0.2g)   Cholesterol 0mg
Protein 2.4g   Sodium 113mg
Carbohydrate 8.1g   Exchange: 1 Vegetable

(Photograph on page 161)

Slicing Green Beans

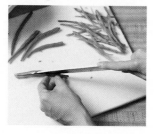

Corn Pudding

Yield: 16 (½-cup) servings

¼ cup granulated sugar substitute (such as Sugar Twin)
¼ cup all-purpose flour
2 teaspoons baking powder
½ teaspoon salt
2 cups fat-free evaporated milk
1½ cups fat-free egg substitute
2 tablespoons margarine, melted
6 cups fresh corn kernels (about 12 ears)
Cooking spray

Combine first 4 ingredients; set aside.

Combine milk, egg substitute, and margarine in a large bowl. Gradually add flour mixture, stirring until smooth. Stir in corn. Pour mixture into a 13- x 9-inch baking dish coated with cooking spray.

Bake, uncovered, at 350° for 40 to 45 minutes or until deep golden and set. Let stand 5 minutes before serving.

Per Serving:

Calories 122	Fiber 2.0g
Fat 2.3g (sat 0.5g)	Cholesterol 2mg
Protein 6.9g	Sodium 243mg
Carbohydrate 20.4g	Exchanges: 1½ Starch, ½ Medium-Fat Meat

If fresh corn is out of season, you can use thawed and drained frozen whole-kernel corn.

Okra-Tomato-Zucchini Medley

Yield: 4 (½-cup) servings

1   small zucchini
Cooking spray
1½ cups sliced fresh okra
2   tablespoons chopped onion
1   cup chopped fresh tomato
⅛   teaspoon dried basil
⅛   teaspoon dried thyme
Dash of freshly ground pepper

Cut zucchini in half lengthwise; cut into ¼-inch-thick slices.

Coat a nonstick skillet with cooking spray; place over medium-high heat until hot. Add zucchini, okra, and onion; sauté 4 minutes.

Stir in tomato and remaining ingredients. Cover and cook over low heat 5 minutes or until thoroughly heated, stirring frequently. Serve immediately.

Per Serving:

Calories 31	**Fiber** 1.3g
Fat 0.4g (sat 0.0g)	**Cholesterol** 0mg
Protein 1.5g	**Sodium** 8mg
Carbohydrate 6.3g	**Exchange:** 1 Vegetable

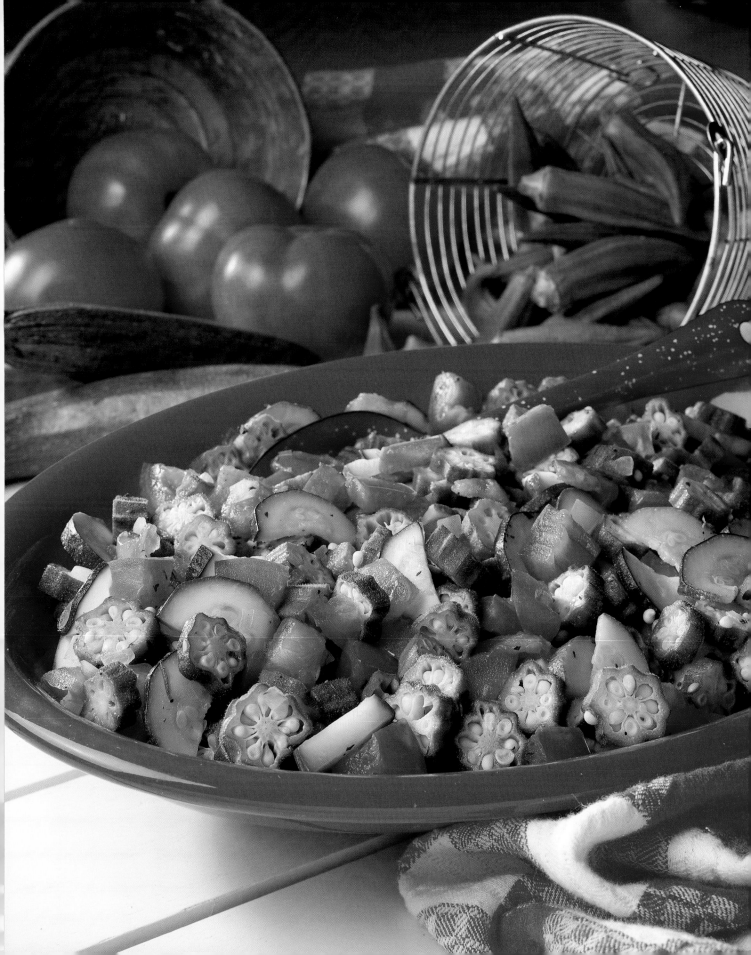

Chili-Fried Potatoes

Yield: 4 servings

3 cups unpeeled, cubed baking potato (about 1 pound)
Olive oil-flavored cooking spray
½ teaspoon olive oil
1 small onion, halved, thinly sliced, and separated into rings
1 teaspoon chili powder
¼ teaspoon salt
½ cup (2 ounces) shredded reduced-fat sharp Cheddar cheese

Arrange potato in a steamer basket over boiling water. Cover and steam 10 minutes or until tender. Remove from heat.

Coat a large nonstick skillet with cooking spray; add oil. Place over medium-high heat until hot. Add onion; sauté 3 minutes or until tender. Add potato, chili powder, and salt. Cook 5 minutes or until potato is lightly browned, stirring often. Sprinkle cheese over potato. Cover, remove from heat, and let stand 1 minute or until cheese melts.

Serve immediately.

Per Serving:

Calories 152	Fiber 2.6g
Fat 3.7g (sat 1.7g)	Cholesterol 10mg
Protein 6.9g	Sodium 263mg
Carbohydrate 23.8g	Exchanges: 1½ Starch, 1 Fat

Just give me a potato, any kind of potato, and I'm happy.

DOLLY PARTON

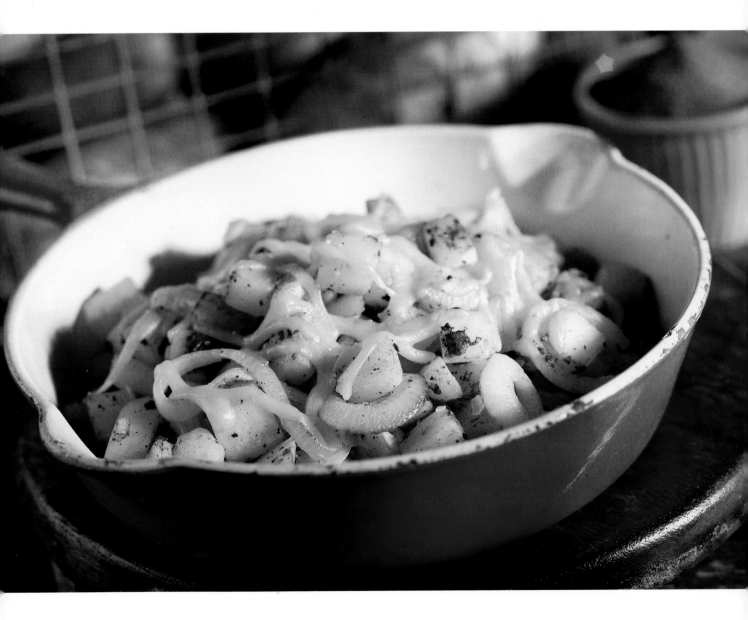

New Potatoes with Chives

Yield: 4 servings

1	pound round red potatoes, quartered
1	teaspoon olive oil
1	tablespoon chopped fresh chives or 1 teaspoon freeze-dried chives
¼	teaspoon salt
⅛	teaspoon pepper

Arrange potato in a steamer basket over boiling water. Cover and steam 17 minutes or until tender.

Place potato in a large bowl. Drizzle with olive oil, and sprinkle with chives, salt, and pepper. Toss well, and serve immediately.

Per Serving:

Calories 94	Fiber 2.1g
Fat 1.2g (sat 0.2g)	Cholesterol 0mg
Protein 2.5g	Sodium 154mg
Carbohydrate 18.9g	Exchange: 1 Starch

Brown Rice Pilaf

Yield: 8 (½-cup) servings

2   cups fat-free, reduced-sodium chicken broth
1   cup brown rice, uncooked
½   cup shredded carrot
½   cup finely chopped celery
½   teaspoon salt
¼   teaspoon ground red pepper
1   clove garlic, minced
¼   cup thinly sliced green onions
3   tablespoons slivered almonds, toasted

Bring broth to a boil in a heavy saucepan; stir in rice and next 5 ingredients.

Cover, reduce heat, and simmer 50 to 55 minutes or until rice is tender and liquid is absorbed. Stir in green onions and almonds.

Serve immediately.

Per Serving:

Calories 117	Fiber 1.6g
Fat 2.6g (sat 0.3g)	Cholesterol 0mg
Protein 2.8g	Sodium 159mg
Carbohydrate 20.2g	Exchanges: 1 Starch, 1 Vegetable, ½ Fat

Southwestern Rice

Yield: 6 (½-cup) servings

1	(16-ounce) can fat-free reduced-sodium chicken broth
1	cup long-grain rice, uncooked
1¼	teaspoons ground cumin
¼	cup thinly sliced green onions

Bring broth to a boil in a large saucepan; add rice and cumin. Return to a boil; cover, reduce heat, and simmer 25 minutes or until rice is tender and liquid is absorbed.

Add green onions; toss gently.

Per Serving:

Calories 122	Fiber 0.5g
Fat 0.3g (sat 0.1g)	Cholesterol 0mg
Protein 2.5g	Sodium 244mg
Carbohydrate 25.7g	Exchanges: 1½ Starch

Vermicelli with Tomato Basil

Yield: 8 (1-cup) servings

8   ounces vermicelli
Cooking spray
2   cloves garlic, minced
1   medium onion, thinly sliced
5   cups peeled, seeded, and chopped tomato (about 5 medium
          tomatoes)
1   (8-ounce) can no-salt-added tomato sauce
¼   cup minced fresh basil
¼   teaspoon salt
⅛   teaspoon pepper
¼   cup freshly grated Parmesan cheese

Cook pasta according to package directions, omitting salt and fat.
Drain.

Coat a Dutch oven with cooking spray; place over medium heat
until hot. Add garlic and onion; sauté 5 minutes or until onion is
tender. Stir in chopped tomato and next 4 ingredients; bring to a
boil. Reduce heat, and simmer, uncovered, 15 minutes, stirring
occasionally.

Add cooked pasta to tomato mixture; cook, uncovered, until mixture is thoroughly heated, stirring occasionally. Sprinkle with
cheese, and serve immediately.

Per Serving:

Calories 163
Fat 1.9g (sat 0.6g)
Protein 6.3g
Carbohydrate 29.9g

Fiber 2.9g
Cholesterol 2mg
Sodium 147mg
Exchanges: 2 Starch

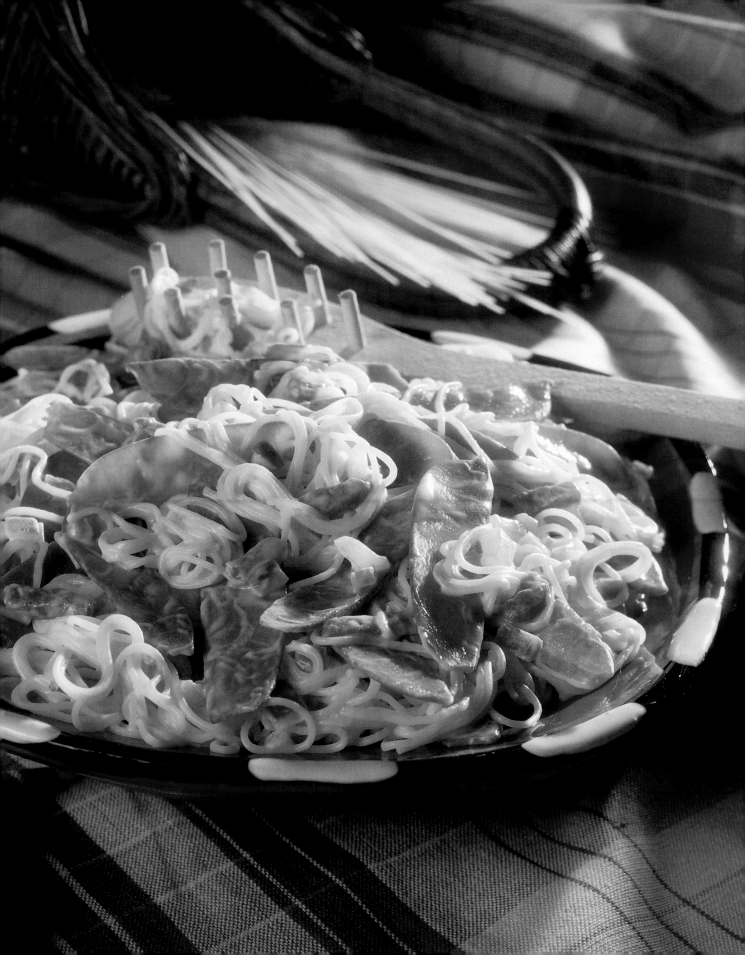

Tangy Dijon Pasta

Yield: 7 (½-cup) servings

4   ounces angel hair pasta, uncooked
2   cups fresh snow pea pods
Cooking spray
½   cup diced purple onion
1   (2-ounce) jar sliced pimiento, drained
¼   cup plus 2 tablespoons low-fat sour cream
3   tablespoons dry white wine or low-sodium chicken broth
2   tablespoons Dijon mustard

Cook pasta according to package directions, omitting salt and fat. Drain and set aside.

Wash peas; trim ends, and remove strings. Cook, uncovered, in a small amount of boiling water 3 minutes. Drain; set aside.

Coat a large skillet with cooking spray; place over medium-high heat until hot. Add onion, and sauté 2 to 3 minutes or until tender. Add pasta, snow peas, and pimiento. Combine sour cream, wine (or broth), and mustard in a small bowl; stir well using a wire whisk. Add sour cream mixture to skillet. Cook, stirring constantly, 2 to 3 minutes or until thoroughly heated. Serve immediately.

Per Serving:

Calories 102	Fiber 1.3g
Fat 2.3g (sat 1.0g)	Cholesterol 5mg
Protein 3.4g	Sodium 137mg
Carbohydrate 16.5g	Exchanges: 1 Starch, ½ Fat

Sausage-Cornbread Dressing

Yield: 12 (¾-cup) servings

2   (7½-ounce) packages yellow corn muffin mix (with egg)
1   cup fat-free milk
Cooking spray
1   pound freshly ground turkey breakfast sausage
2   cups chopped onion (about 2 medium)
1¾   cups chopped celery (about 5 stalks)
3   cups white bread cubes, toasted
2   teaspoons rubbed sage
1   teaspoon pepper
4   cups fat-free, reduced-sodium chicken broth
½   cup fat-free egg substitute

Prepare muffin mix according to package directions for cornbread, using fat-free milk. Let cool; crumble and set aside.

Coat a large nonstick skillet with cooking spray. Place over medium heat until hot. Add sausage, onion, and celery; cook until sausage is browned and vegetables are tender. stirring until sausage crumbles. Drain and pat dry with paper towels.

Combine cornbread, bread cubes, sage, and pepper in a large bowl; stir in sausage mixture. Add chicken broth and egg substitute, stirring well. Spoon mixture into a 13- x 9-inch baking dish coated with cooking spray.

Bake, uncovered, at 350° for 1 hour or until browned. Serve warm.

Per Serving:

Calories 143	Fiber 1.2g
Fat 5.3g (sat 3.0g)	Cholesterol 24mg
Protein 9.6g	Sodium 501mg
Carbohydrate 13.8g	Exchanges: 1 Starch, 1 Medium-Fat Meat

Soups & Sandwiches

Easy Weeknight Chili, page 190

Potato-Corn Chowder

Yield: 5 (1½-cup) servings

Cooking spray
¾   cup chopped green pepper
⅓   cup chopped onion
2¾   cups fat-free, reduced-sodium chicken broth
2   cups chopped red potato
½   teaspoon salt
¼   teaspoon pepper
¼   cup cornstarch
2¼   cups fat-free milk
2¼   cups frozen whole-kernel corn
1   (2-ounce) jar diced pimiento, drained

Coat a medium saucepan with cooking spray; place over medium-high heat until hot. Add chopped green pepper and onion; sauté 5 minutes or until tender. Stir in broth and next 3 ingredients. Bring to a boil; reduce heat, and simmer, uncovered, 6 to 8 minutes or until potato is tender.

Combine cornstarch and milk, stirring until smooth; gradually add to potato mixture, stirring constantly. Stir in corn and diced pimiento; bring to a boil over medium heat, stirring constantly. Cook, stirring constantly, 1 minute or until mixture is thickened. Serve immediately.

Per Serving:

Calories 167	Fiber 2.6g
Fat 0.9g (sat 0.2g)	Cholesterol 2mg
Protein 8.4g	Sodium 606mg
Carbohydrate 33.5g	Exchanges: 2 Starch, 1 Vegetable

French Onion Soup

Yield: 8 (1½-cup) servings

Cooking spray
2 tablespoons reduced-calorie margarine
6 large onions (about 3 pounds), cut into ¼-inch-thick slices
2 (10½-ounce) cans beef consommé, undiluted
1 (14¼-ounce) can no-salt-added beef broth
1⅓ cups water
¼ teaspoon pepper
¼ cup dry white wine
8 (1-inch) slices French bread
¼ cup grated Parmesan cheese

Coat a large Dutch oven with cooking spray; add margarine. Place over medium-high heat until margarine melts. Add onion; sauté 5 minutes. Stir in consommé, broth, water, and pepper; bring to a boil. Reduce heat, and simmer, uncovered, 35 minutes. Add wine, and simmer, uncovered, 5 minutes.

Place bread on a baking sheet; sprinkle with cheese. Broil 3 inches from heat until cheese is golden. Ladle soup evenly into bowls; top each serving with a bread slice.

Per Serving:

Calories 177	Fiber 2.8g
Fat 3.6g (sat 0.9g)	Cholesterol 17mg
Protein 8.0g	Sodium 710mg
Carbohydrate 27.1g	Exchanges: 2 Starch, ½ Fat

To make a good soup, the pot
must only simmer or "smile."

French proverb

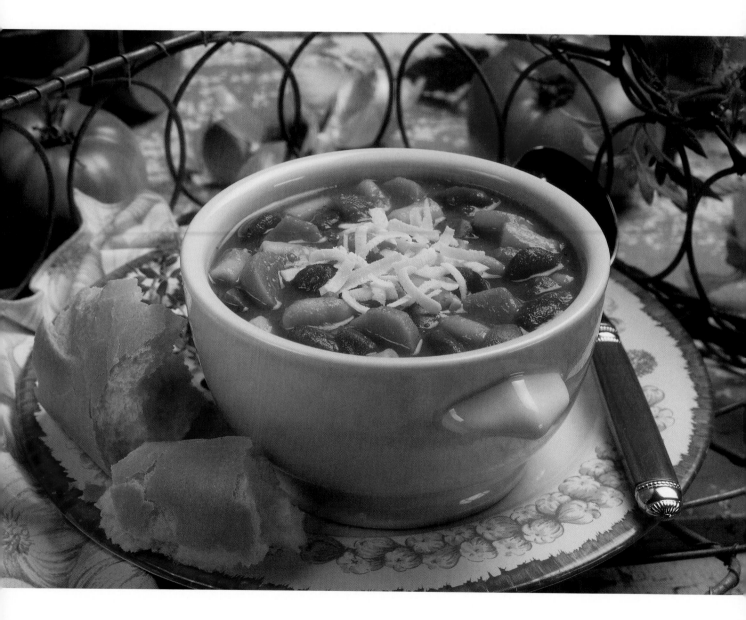

Italian Pasta and Bean Soup

Yield: 8 (1 ¼-cup) servings

Cooking spray
1   tablespoon olive oil
1   cup chopped onion
1   cup sliced carrot
½   cup chopped green pepper
2   cloves garlic, crushed
2   (14¼-ounce) cans no-salt-added beef broth
1   (28-ounce) can crushed tomatoes
1   (15-ounce) can cannellini beans, rinsed and drained
1   (15-ounce) can red kidney beans, rinsed and drained
1½   teaspoons dried Italian seasoning
½   teaspoon salt
¼   teaspoon pepper
6   ounces ditalini pasta
½   cup freshly grated Parmesan cheese

Coat a large Dutch oven with cooking spray; add oil and place over medium-high heat. Add onion and next 3 ingredients; sauté until vegetables are crisp-tender.

Add beef broth and next 6 ingredients; bring to a boil. Cover, reduce heat, and simmer 20 minutes, stirring occasionally.

Add pasta to vegetable mixture. Cover and cook 10 to 15 minutes or until pasta is tender. Ladle soup into individual bowls; top each serving with 1 tablespoon cheese.

Per Serving:

Calories 232	Fiber 4.2g
Fat 4.5g (sat 1.5g)	Cholesterol 5mg
Protein 10.8g	Sodium 497mg
Carbohydrate 36.2g	Exchanges: 2 Starch, 1 Vegetable, ½ High-Fat Meat

Chunky Chicken Noodle Soup

Yield: 6 (1-cup) servings

1   (3-pound) broiler-fryer, cut up and skinned
4   cups water
¾   teaspoon poultry seasoning
¼   teaspoon dried thyme
3   celery tops
2   cups water
1   cup medium egg noodles, uncooked
½   cup sliced celery
½   cup sliced carrot
⅓   cup sliced green onions
2   tablespoons minced fresh parsley
2   teaspoons chicken-flavored bouillon granules
¼   teaspoon coarsely ground pepper
1   bay leaf
Additional coarsely ground pepper (optional)

Combine first 5 ingredients in a Dutch oven; bring to a boil. Cover, reduce heat, and simmer 45 minutes or until chicken is tender. Remove chicken from broth, discarding celery and reserving broth.

Skim fat from broth. Add 2 cups water and next 8 ingredients to broth; bring to a boil. Cover, reduce heat, and simmer 20 minutes.

Bone and chop chicken; add to broth mixture. Cook 5 minutes or until thoroughly heated. Discard bay leaf. Ladle soup into bowls, and sprinkle with additional pepper, if desired.

Per Serving:

Calories 204	Fiber 1.0g
Fat 6.9g (sat 1.9g)	Cholesterol 82mg
Protein 25.4g	Sodium 358mg
Carbohydrate 9.1g	Exchanges: 1 Starch, 3 Lean Meat

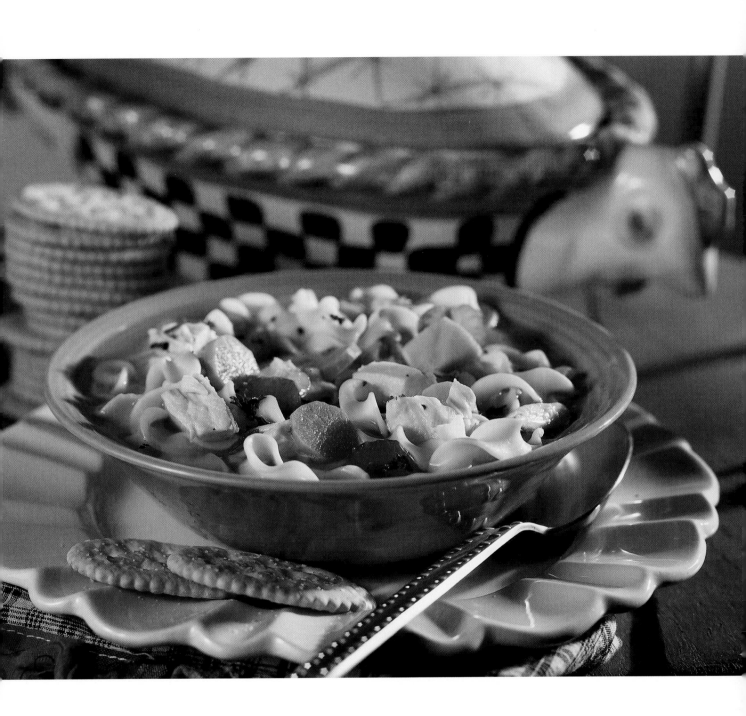

Worries go down better with soup.

Yiddish proverb

Spicy Ham and Bean Soup

Yield: 10 (1½-cup) servings

1	pound dried Great Northern beans
4	quarts water
1	pound reduced-salt lean ham, cubed
2¾	cups chopped red potato (about 4 medium)
1¾	cups chopped onion (about 2 medium)
1	cup chopped carrot (about 1 large)
¾	cup chopped celery (about 2 stalks)
1	(5.5-ounce) can spicy vegetable juice
1	(4.5-ounce) can chopped green chiles, undrained
1	tablespoon chopped pickled jalapeño pepper
1	tablespoon pickled jalapeño pepper juice
1	tablespoon low-sodium Worcestershire sauce
½	teaspoon garlic powder
½	teaspoon chili powder

Sort and wash beans; place in a large Dutch oven. Add water; cover and let stand 2 hours.

Bring bean mixture to a boil; reduce heat, and simmer, uncovered, 1 hour. Add ham and next 4 ingredients; bring to a boil. Reduce heat, and simmer, uncovered, 1 hour.

Add vegetable juice and remaining ingredients; bring to a boil. Reduce heat, and simmer, uncovered, 1 hour or until beans are tender and soup is thickened.

Per Serving:

Calories 255	**Fiber** 20.1g
Fat 3.0g (sat 1.0g)	**Cholesterol** 19mg
Protein 16.9g	**Sodium** 427mg
Carbohydrate 41.4g	**Exchanges:** 2 Starch, 2 Vegetable, 1 Lean Meat

White Bean Chili

Yield: 4 (1½-cup) servings

Cooking spray
1   cup chopped onion (about 1 medium)
1   clove garlic, minced
2   (15-ounce) cans cannellini beans, drained and divided
1   (4-ounce) can chopped green chiles, undrained
2¼ cups fat-free, reduced-sodium chicken broth
1½ cups chopped cooked chicken (skinned before cooking and cooked
        without salt)
1   teaspoon chili powder
⅛   teaspoon salt

Coat a large saucepan with cooking spray; place over medium-high heat until hot. Add onion and garlic; sauté until tender. Add 1 can beans and next 5 ingredients.

Mash remaining 1 can beans with a fork; add to chicken mixture in saucepan. Bring to a boil; cover, reduce heat, and simmer 20 minutes.

Per Serving:

Calories 207	**Fiber** 3.3g
Fat 4.3g (sat 1.0g)	**Cholesterol** 43mg
Protein 19.4g	**Sodium** 554mg
Carbohydrate 19.6g	**Exchanges:** 1 Starch, 1 Vegetable, 2 Lean Meat

Easy Weeknight Chili

Yield: 6 (1½-cup) servings

Cooking spray
1   pound ground round
1¼   cups chopped onion (about 1 large)
1¼   cups chopped green pepper (about 2 small)
6   cloves garlic, minced
2   (14½-ounce) cans no-salt-added stewed tomatoes,
          undrained and chopped
1   (15-ounce) can no-salt-added kidney beans, drained
1   (8-ounce) can no-salt-added tomato sauce
1   (1-ounce) envelope onion soup mix
1   cup water
3   tablespoons chili powder
1   tablespoon paprika
1¼   teaspoons hot sauce
6   tablespoons (1½-ounces) shredded reduced-fat sharp Cheddar cheese

Coat a Dutch oven with cooking spray; Place over medium-high heat until hot. Add meat and next 3 ingredients; cook until meat is browned, stirring until it crumbles. Drain.

Return mixture to Dutch oven; add tomatoes and next 7 ingredients. Bring to a boil; cover, reduce heat, and simmer 20 minutes, stirring occasionally. To serve, ladle chili into six bowls; top each with 1 tablespoon cheese.

Per Serving:

Calories 302	Fiber 9.5g
Fat 6.6g (sat 2.2g)	Cholesterol 52mg
Protein 29.0g	Sodium 277mg
Carbohydrate 34.7g	Exchanges: 2 Starch, 1 Vegetable, 3 Lean Meat

(Photograph on page 181)

Veggie Melts

Yield: 2 servings (serving size: 2 muffin halves)

⅔ cup thinly sliced cucumber
½ cup shredded carrot
2 tablespoons sliced green onions
2 tablespoons fat-free Italian dressing
½ cup (2 ounces) shredded part-skim mozzarella cheese
2 English muffins, split and toasted
¼ cup alfalfa sprouts

Combine first 4 ingredients; set aside.

Sprinkle cheese evenly over muffin halves. Broil 5½ inches from heat 1 minute or until cheese melts.

Top muffin halves evenly with cucumber mixture and sprouts. Serve immediately.

Per Serving:

Calories 274	Fiber 3.0g
Fat 6.0g (sat 3.2g)	Cholesterol 16mg
Protein 13.1g	Sodium 639mg
Carbohydrate 41.9g	Exchanges: 2 Starch, 2 Vegetable, 1 Medium-Fat Meat

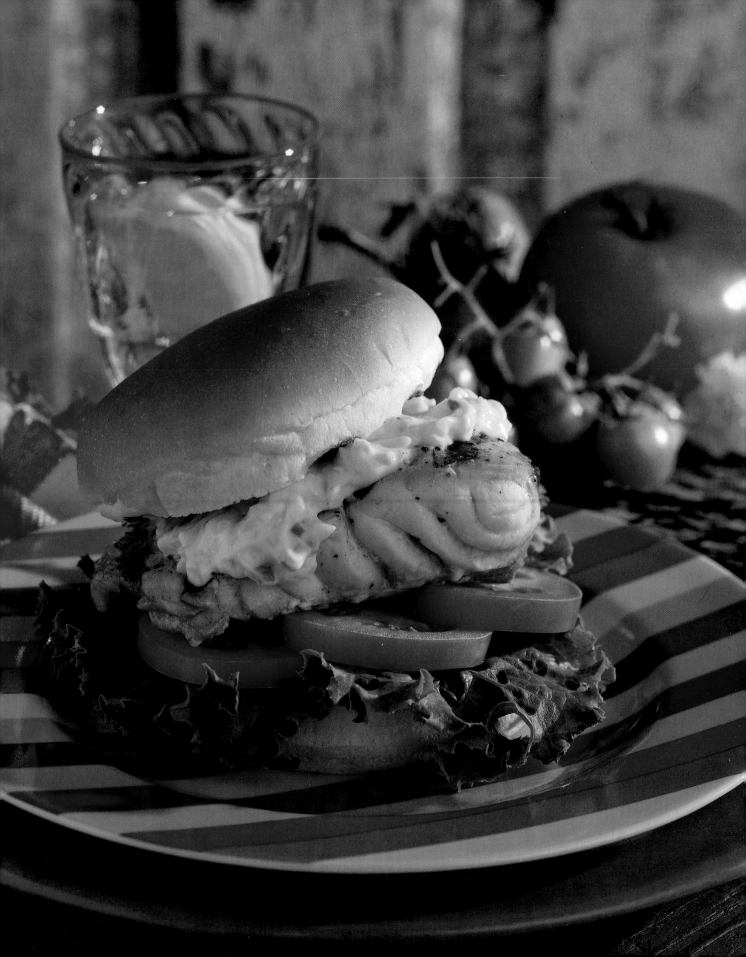

Tangy Grouper Sandwiches

Yield: 4 servings

2	tablespoons lemon juice
1	teaspoon low-sodium Worcestershire sauce
1	teaspoon olive oil
½	teaspoon pepper
⅛	teaspoon paprika
3	tablespoons nonfat mayonnaise
1	tablespoon minced onion
2	teaspoons dill pickle relish
½	teaspoon prepared mustard
Cooking spray	
1	(1-pound) grouper fillet, cut into 4 pieces
4	green leaf lettuce leaves
12	(¼-inch-thick) slices plum tomato
4	hamburger buns, split and toasted

Combine first 5 ingredients; set aside. Combine mayonnaise and next 3 ingredients; set aside.

Coat grill rack with cooking spray; place on grill over medium-hot coals (350° to 400°). Place fish on rack; grill, covered, 5 minutes on each side or until fish flakes easily when tested with a fork, basting with lemon juice mixture.

Layer 1 lettuce leaf, 3 slices tomato, and 1 piece fish on bottom half of each bun. Spoon mayonnaise mixture evenly onto fish, and cover with top halves of buns. Serve immediately.

Per Serving:

Calories 243	Fiber 1.0g
Fat 5.3g (sat 0.8g)	Cholesterol 52mg
Protein 25.0g	Sodium 338mg
Carbohydrate 22.6g	Exchanges: 1½ Starch, 3 Very Lean Meat

Asian Chicken Pitas

Yield: 2 servings

2	(4-ounce) skinned and boned chicken breast halves
½	cup bean sprouts
¼	cup diced water chestnuts
¼	cup sliced green onions
1	tablespoon rice vinegar
1	tablespoon low-sodium soy sauce
1	teaspoon sesame oil
1	(7-inch) whole wheat pita bread round, cut in half crosswise
2	lettuce leaves

Place chicken in a medium saucepan; add water to cover. Bring to a boil. Reduce heat to medium, and cook, uncovered, 15 minutes or until chicken is done. Drain. Let chicken cool to touch. Chop chicken into bite-size pieces.

Combine chicken, bean sprouts, water chestnuts, and green onions. Combine vinegar, soy sauce, and oil; pour over chicken mixture, tossing gently.

Line each pita half with one lettuce leaf; spoon chicken mixture evenly into pita halves.

Per Serving:

Calories 271	**Fiber** 3.4g
Fat 5.9g (sat fat 1.2g)	**Cholesterol** 70mg
Protein 28.2g	**Sodium** 264mg
Carbohydrate 22.4g	**Exchanges:** 1½ Starch, 3½ Very Lean Meat

Turkey Reubens

Yield: 6 servings

1½ cups finely shredded cabbage
1½ tablespoons fat-free Thousand Island dressing
1 tablespoon reduced-fat mayonnaise
1 tablespoon Dijon mustard
12 (1-ounce) slices rye bread
6 ounces thinly sliced cooked turkey breast
6 (¾-ounce) slices reduced-fat Swiss cheese
Butter-flavored cooking spray

Combine first 3 ingredients in a medium bowl; toss well, and set aside.

Spread mustard evenly over 6 bread slices, and top with turkey. Top each with 1 cheese slice and ¼ cup cabbage mixture. Top with remaining bread slices.

Spray both sides of each sandwich with cooking spray; place on a hot griddle or skillet coated with cooking spray. Cook 2 minutes on each side or until bread is lightly browned and cheese melts. Serve immediately.

Per Serving:

Calories 274	**Fiber** 3.9g
Fat 7.1g (sat 2.7g)	**Cholesterol** 34mg
Protein 21.0g	**Sodium** 497mg
Carbohydrate 32.4g	**Exchanges:** 2 Starch, 1 Vegetable, 2 Lean Meat

Taco Burgers

Yield: 4 servings

¾   pound ground round
½   cup salsa, divided
Cooking spray
½   cup canned fat-free refried beans
4   reduced-calorie whole wheat hamburger buns
1   cup shredded lettuce
½   cup chopped tomato
½   cup (2 ounces) shredded reduced-fat sharp Cheddar cheese

Combine meat and ¼ cup salsa. Shape meat mixture into 4 (½-inch-thick) patties. Coat a nonstick skillet with cooking spray. Place over medium heat until hot. Add patties, and cook 4 to 5 minutes on each side or until done. Remove from skillet; drain on paper towels.

Spread 2 tablespoons refried beans on bottom half of each bun. Top each with ¼ cup shredded lettuce, 2 tablespoons chopped tomato, and 2 tablespoons shredded cheese. Top each with a meat patty. Spoon remaining ¼ cup salsa evenly over patties. Top with remaining bun halves.

Per Serving:

Calories 296	**Fiber** 3.4g
Fat 9.6g (sat 3.4g)	**Cholesterol** 62mg
Protein 26.2g	**Sodium** 567mg
Carbohydrate 24.1g	**Exchanges:** 1½ Starch, 3 Lean Meat

This sandwich tastes like a taco but looks like a hamburger. And you can have it on the table in less time than it takes to go to a fast-food drive-through.

Stromboli

Yield: 5 servings

Cooking spray
½   cup chopped onion
1   (10-ounce) can refrigerated pizza crust dough
2   tablespoons coarse-grained mustard
1   cup (4 ounces) shredded part-skim mozzarella cheese
6   ounces thinly sliced reduced-fat, low-salt ham
1   teaspoon dried Italian seasoning

Coat a small nonstick skillet with cooking spray; place over medium-high heat until hot. Add onion; sauté 4 minutes.

Unroll dough on a baking sheet coated with cooking spray; press into a 12- x 8-inch rectangle. Spread mustard over dough to within ½ inch of edges. Arrange cheese, onion, and ham lengthwise down the center of dough, leaving a ½-inch border at both ends (Step 1). Sprinkle seasoning over ham. At 1-inch intervals on long sides of rectangle, cut slits from edge of ham to edge of dough (Step 2). Alternating sides, fold strips at an angle across filling (Step 3). Coat top of dough with cooking spray. Bake at 425° for 12 minutes or until browned.

Per Serving:

Calories 258	**Fiber** 1.2g
Fat 8.1g (sat 3.2g)	**Cholesterol** 30mg
Protein 17.0g	**Sodium** 763mg
Carbohydrate 29.3g	**Exchanges:** 2 Starch, 1½ Medium-Fat Meat

Making a Stromboli Sandwich

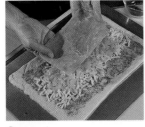

Step 1

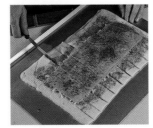

Step 2

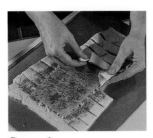

Step 3

7-DAY MENU PLANNER

Explanation of Menus

Use these menus and the recipes in the book to make your meal plan work for you. Since meal and snack plans differ according to dietary treatments and goals, this weekly menu planner is simply a guide to recipes and food items that make pleasing meals. Use your own meal plan to determine the number of servings you can have, or the number of other items you can add to your meal.

Page numbers are provided for you to refer to the recipes in the book. The other items are listed to round out the meal; substitute as desired. Start with this menu plan for ideas and then create your own meal plans using other recipes in the book.

Day 1

BREAKFAST
Corn flakes cereal
Banana
Fat-free milk

LUNCH
Shrimp Salad (page 157)
Whole wheat roll
Tomato slices
Cantaloupe wedge

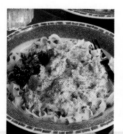

DINNER
Turkey Stroganoff (page 135)
Steamed green beans
Unsweetened applesauce

SNACK
No-sugar-added ice cream

Day 2

BREAKFAST
Reduced-fat frozen waffles with sugar-free syrup
Fresh strawberries
Fat-free milk

LUNCH
Sun-Dried Tomato Pizza (page 85)
Carrot sticks
Fresh fruit salad (grapes, cantaloupe, pineapple)

DINNER
Greek-Style Flounder (page 66)
Marinated Tomato Slices (page 153)
Whole wheat rolls

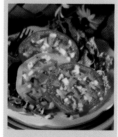

SNACK
Reduced-fat Cheddar cheese
Rice cakes

Day 3

BREAKFAST
Reduced-fat biscuit (canned)
Turkey sausage
Orange juice
Fat-free milk

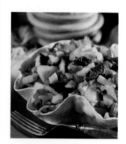

LUNCH
Chicken Taco Salad (page 159)
Orange

DINNER
Thin-Crust Vegetable Pizza (page 86)
Tossed salad with low-fat dressing
No-sugar-added ice cream

SNACK
Peanut butter
Saltine crackers

Day 4	Day 5	Day 6	Day 7

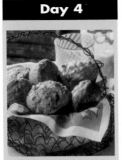

BREAKFAST
Whole Wheat Banana Muffins (page 32)
Fresh strawberries
Fat-free milk

LUNCH
Pizza Pockets (page 87)
Carrot sticks
Grapes

DINNER
Lemon-Roasted Chicken (page 133)
Steamed broccoli
Brown rice
Holiday Cranberry Salad (page 140)

SNACK
Chocolate-Peppermint Cookies (page 52)
Fat-free milk

BREAKFAST
Whole wheat
   English muffins
Poached egg
Grapefruit half

LUNCH
Chicken and Fettuccine Salad (page 160)
Breadsticks
Apple

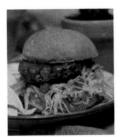

DINNER
Taco Burgers (page 196)
Low-fat tortilla chips
Citrus fruit salad
   (pineapple and
   orange segments)

SNACK
Marinated Cheese Appetizers (page 19)

BREAKFAST
Whole wheat toast
   with low-sugar
   jelly
Scrambled egg or
   egg substitute
Orange juice
Fat-free milk

LUNCH
Turkey Reubens (page 195)
Low-fat potato chips
Banana

DINNER
Vegetable Lasagna (page 90)
Tossed salad with
   low-fat dressing
Sugar-free gelatin
   dessert

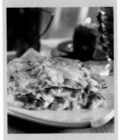

SNACK
Peanut Butter Ice Cream Sandwiches (page 46)

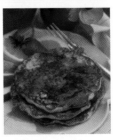

BREAKFAST
Applesauce Pancakes (page 37)
Grapefruit juice
Fat-free milk

LUNCH
White Bean Chili (page 189)
Low-fat tortilla chips
Pineapple slices

DINNER
Lamb Shish Kabobs (page 108)
Rice
French bread

SNACK
Spicy Snack Mix (page 16)
Fat-free milk

Nutrition Notes

Delicious Ways to Control Diabetes gives you the nutrition facts you want to know. We provide the following information with every recipe.

values are for one serving of the recipe

Per Serving:

Calories 299

Fat 2.0g (sat 0.4g)

Protein 22.8g

Carbohydrate 29.1g

total carbohydrate in one serving

Fiber 2.0 g

grams are abbreviated "g"

Cholesterol 47 mg

milligrams are abbreviated "mg"

Sodium 644mg

Exchanges: 2 Starch, 2 Medium-Fat Meat

exchange values are for one serving

Nutritional Analyses

The nutritional values used in our calculations either come from a computer program by Computrition, Inc., or are provided by food manufacturers. The values are based on the following assumptions:

- When we give a range for an ingredient, we calculate using the lesser amount.
- Only the amount of marinade absorbed is calculated.
- Garnishes and optional ingredients are not included in the analysis.

Diabetic Exchanges

Exchange values for all recipes are provided for people who use them for meal planning. The exchange values are based on the *Exchange Lists for Meal Planning* developed by the American Diabetes Association and The American Dietetic Association.

Carbohydrates

If you count carbohydrates, look for the value in the nutrient analysis. New guidelines from the American Diabetes Association loosen the restriction on sugar and suggest that it's the total amount of carbohydrate instead of the *type* of carbohydrate that affects blood glucose. We have used small amounts of sugar in some recipes. We've also used a variety of sugar substitutes when the use of a sugar substitute yields a quality product.

Sodium

Current dietary recommendations advise a daily sodium intake of 2,400 milligrams. We have limited the sodium in these recipes by using reduced-sodium products whenever possible.

If you must restrict sodium in your diet, please note the sodium value per serving and see if you should modify the recipe further.

Recipe Index

See page 206 for Quick and Easy
Recipe lists.

Quick and Easy Recipes

Metric Equivalents

The recipes that appear in this cookbook use the standard United States method for measuring liquid and dry or solid ingredients (teaspoons, tablespoons, and cups). The information in the following charts is provided to help cooks outside the U.S. successfully use these recipes. All equivalents are approximate.

Equivalents for Different Types of Ingredients

A standard cup measure of a dry or solid ingredient will vary in weight depending on the type of ingredient. A standard cup of liquid is the same volume for any type of liquid. Use the following chart when converting standard cup measures to grams (weight) or milliliters (volume).

Standard Cup	Fine Powder (ex. flour)	Grain (ex. rice)	Granular (ex. sugar)	Liquid Solids (ex. butter)	Liquid (ex. milk)
1	140 g	150 g	190 g	200 g	240 ml
¾	105 g	113 g	143 g	150 g	180 ml
⅔	93 g	100 g	125 g	133 g	160 ml
½	70 g	75 g	95 g	100 g	120 ml
⅓	47 g	50 g	63 g	67 g	80 ml
¼	35 g	38 g	48 g	50 g	60 ml
⅛	18 g	19 g	24 g	25 g	30 ml

Dry Ingredients by Weight

(To convert ounces to grams, multiply the number of ounces by 30.)

1 oz	=	1/16 lb	=	30 g
4 oz	=	¼ lb	=	120 g
8 oz	=	½ lb	=	240 g
12 oz	=	¾ lb	=	360 g
16 oz	=	1 lb	=	480 g

Length

(To convert inches to centimeters, multiply the number of inches by 2.5.)

1 in	=				=	2.5 cm	
6 in	=	½ ft			=	15 cm	
12 in	=	1 ft			=	30 cm	
36 in	=	3 ft	=	1 yd	=	90 cm	
40 in	=				=	100 cm	= 1 m

Liquid Ingredients by Volume

¼ tsp						1 ml	
½ tsp						2 ml	
1 tsp						5 ml	
3 tsp	=	1 tbls		=	½ fl oz	=	15 ml
		2 tbls	=	⅛ cup	=	1 fl oz	=	30 ml
		4 tbls	=	¼ cup	=	2 fl oz	=	60 ml
		5⅓ tbls	=	⅓ cup	=	3 fl oz	=	80 ml
		8 tbls	=	½ cup	=	4 fl oz	=	120 ml
		10⅔ tbls	=	⅔ cup	=	5 fl oz	=	160 ml
		12 tbls	=	¾ cup	=	6 fl oz	=	180 ml
		16 tbls	=	1 cup	=	8 fl oz	=	240 ml
		1 pt	=	2 cups	=	16 fl oz	=	480 ml
		1 qt	=	4 cups	=	32 fl oz	=	960 ml
					33 fl oz	=	1000 ml = 1 liter

Cooking/Oven Temperatures

	Fahrenheit	Celsius	Gas Mark
Freeze Water	32° F	0° C	
Room Temperature	68° F	20° C	
Boil Water	212° F	100° C	
Bake	325° F	160° C	3
	350° F	180° C	4
	375° F	190° C	5
	400° F	200° C	6
	425° F	220° C	7
	450° F	230° C	8
Broil			Grill

Good News About Diabetes!

Try the positive new magazine filled with upbeat information and inspiration for happier, healthier living

Here's what you'll get...

- Delicious recipes with exchanges
- Mouthwatering, full-color photography
- New products and latest research
- Support for spouses and family
- Motivational stories from others living with diabetes
- All approved by a medical board of diabetes experts

Plus, a portion of all proceeds will be donated to diabetes research!

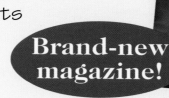

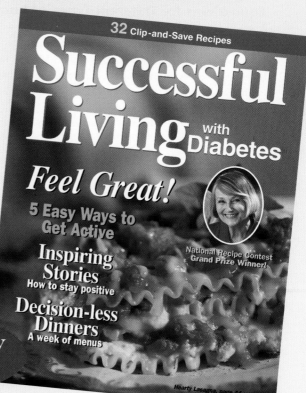

Get your FREE preview issue today!

To get your free preview issue please write to:

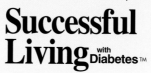

Successful Living with Diabetes™

P.O. Box 420235 • Palm Coast, FL 32142-0235 • or call 1-800-829-9097